T0231377

Faith-Based Social Services:
Measures, Assessments,
and Effectiveness

Faith-Based Social Services: Measures, Assessments, and Effectiveness has been co-published simultaneously as *Journal of Religion & Spirituality in Social Work*, Volume 25, Numbers 3/4 2006.

Monographic Separates from the *Journal of Religion & Spirituality in Social Work*™

For additional information on these and other Haworth Press titles, including descriptions, tables of contents, reviews, and prices, use the QuickSearch

Faith-Based Social Services: Measures, Assessments, and Effectiveness, edited by Stephanie C. Boddie and Ram A. Cnaan (Vol. 25, No. ¾, 2006). *Read the latest studies on the effectiveness of religious-based services–and the problems revealed in the assessment.*

Social Work and Divinity, edited by Daniel Lee, DSW, and Robert O'Gorman, PhD (Vol. 24, No. 1/2, 2005). *"Diverse, fascinating, and thought-provoking. . . . Explores theoretical and practical aspects of dual degree programs and other structures for relating the two professions. It will help nourish the transitional space between social work and divinity. With chapters ranging from conceptual to programmatic to empirical, the collection seems especially enriching for boundary spanners who have feet in both camps but who often work at the boundary alone." (Terry A. Wolfer, PhD, Associate Professor, College of Social Work, University of South Carolina)*

Criminal Justice: Retribution vs. Restoration, edited by Eleanor Hannon Judah, DSW, ACSW, and Rev. Michael Bryant, PhD (Vol. 23, No. 1/2, 2004). *"Timely and necessary. . . . Of interest to students of social, economic, and behavioral sciences, philosophy, theology, and cultural history, as well as to the general public. As a student and teacher of social policy, social justice, and human development. I find this book thought provoking and I will recommend it to my students." (David G. Gil, DSW, Professor of Social Policy, Heller School for Social Policy and Management, Brandeis University)*

Practicing Social Justice, edited by John J. Stretch, PhD, MBA, ACSW, LCSW, Ellen M. Burkemper, PhD, LCSW, MFT, William J. Hutchison, PhD, and Jan Wilson, ACSW, LCSW (Vol. 22, No. 2/3, 2003). *"I highly recommend this important edited work to practitioners, academics, and students majoring in the human services and related fields. . . . Fills an important void in the area of social justice and related issues. . . . Offers a detailed analysis of numerous social justice issues." (John T. Pardeck, PhD, LCSW, Editor,* Journal of Social Work in Disability and Rehabilitation*)*

*Issues in Global Aging,** edited by Frederick L. Ahearn, Jr., DSW (Vol. 20, No. 3/4, 2001). *"Fine scholarship . . . very useful. Ahearn has assembled a fine cohort of experts on aging who address various issues. The first section approaches them from the western industrial model perspective, but also provides an example of an Islamic traditional approach. The second section deals less with formal religiosity than with issues of spiritual transcendence in older persons. A balanced portrait of the aged as people rather than statistics." (Charles Guzzetta, EdD, Professor, Hunter College, City University of New York)*

*Transpersonal Perspectives on Spirituality in Social Work,** edited by Edward R. Canda, PhD, and Elizabeth D. Smith, DSW (Vol. 20, No. ½, 2001). *"Comprehensive . . . provides theoretical and practice-oriented studies on the emerging field of Transpersonal social work. The writing is both scholarly and relevant to practice. Of interest to scholars, practitioners, and students alike." (John R. Graham, PhD, RSW, Associate Professor, Faculty of Social Work, University of Calgary, Alberta, Canada)*

*Raising Our Children Out of Poverty,** edited by John J. Stretch, PhD, Maria Bartlett, PhD, William J. Hutchison, PhD, Susan A. Taylor, PhD, and Jan Wilson, MSW (Vol. 19, No. 2, 1999). *This book shows what can be done at the national and local community levels to raise children out of poverty by strengthening families, communities, and social services.*

*Postmodernism, Religion and the Future of Social Work,** edited by Roland G. Meinert, PhD, John T. Pardeck, PhD, and John W. Murphy, PhD (Vol. 18, No. 3, 1998). *"Critically important for social work as it attempts to effectively respond to its increasingly complex roles and demands. . . . A book worth owning and studying." (John M. Herrick, PhD, Acting Director, School of Social Work, Michigan State University, East Lansing, Michigan)*

Spirituality in Social Work: New Directions,* edited by Edward R. Canda, PhD (Vol. 18, No. 2, 1998). *"Provides interesting insights and references for those who seek to develop curricula responsive to the spiritual challenges confronting our profession and the populations we serve."* (Au-Deane S. Cowley, PhD, Associate Dean, Graduate School of Social Work, University of Utah, Salt Lake City)

Faith-Based Social Services: Measures, Assessments, and Effectiveness

Stephanie C. Boddie
Ram A. Cnaan
Editors

Faith-Based Social Services: Measures, Assessments, and Effectiveness has been co-published simultaneously as *Journal of Religion & Spirituality in Social Work*, Volume 25, Numbers 3/4 2006.

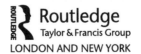

Routledge
Taylor & Francis Group
LONDON AND NEW YORK

First published 2006 by The Haworth Press, Inc
10 Alice Street, Binghamton, NY 13904-1580

This edition published in 2012 by Routledge
2 Park Square, Milton Park, Abingdon, Oxon OX14 4RN
711 Third Avenue, New York, NY 10017, USA
Routledge is an imprint of the Taylor & Francis Group, an informa business

Faith-Based Social Services: Measures, Assessments, and Effectiveness has been co-published simultaneously as *Journal of Religion & Spirituality in Social Work*, Volume 25, Numbers 3/4 2006.

Library of Congress Cataloging-in-Publication Data

Faith-based social services : measures, assessments, and effectiveness / Stephanie C. Boddie, Ram A. Cnaan, editors.
    p. cm.
    "Co-published simultaneously as Journal of Religion & Spirituality in Social Work, Volume 25, Numbers 3/4 2006."
    Includes bibliographical references and index.
    ISBN-13: 978-0-7890-3523-3 (hard cover)
    ISBN-10: 0-7890-3523-5 (hard cover)
    ISBN-13: 978-0-7890-3524-0 (soft cover)
    ISBN-10: 0-7890-3524-3 (soft cover)
    1. Faith-based human services–United States–Evaluation. I. Boddie, Stephanie C. II. Cnaan, Ram A. III. Journal of religion & spirituality in social work.
HV530.F35.2007
361.7'50973–dc22
                                   2006030418

Faith-Based Social Services: Measures, Assessments, and Effectiveness

CONTENTS

SECTION II: EMERGING EMPIRICAL FINDINGS

ABOUT THE EDITORS

Stephanie C. Boddie, PhD, is Assistant Professor at the George Warren Brown School of Social Work at Washington University in St. Louis and Faculty Associate at the Center for Social Development. She is also a non-resident Fellow at the Program for Research on Religion and Urban Civil Society and the Program for Organized Religion and Social Work at the University of Pennsylvania. Her work as lead consultant for the Annie E. Casey Foundation's Faith and Families Portfolio provides a unique perspective to her academic work. She was the Co-Principal Investigator for the Philadelphia Census of Congregations and their Social and Community Services. She has developed courses, seminars, and workshops to equip social workers, community leaders, and faith leaders to partner to develop community-based programs. She is also the co-author of *The Newer Deal: Social Work and Religion in Partnership, The Invisible Caring Hand: American Congregations and the Provision of Welfare*, and *The Other Philadelphia Story: How Local Congregations Support Quality of Life in Urban America*. Dr. Boddie had also written over 20 book chapters, articles, and reports on faith-based services, asset-based community development, and civic service.

Ram A. Cnaan, PhD, is Professor and Associate Dean for research, and Chair of the Doctoral Program in Social Welfare at the University of Pennsylvania, School of Social Policy & Practice. He is also Director of the Program for Religion and Social Policy Research (PRSPR) at the University of Pennsylvania, School of Social Policy & Practice. He conducted one of the first national studies on the role of local religious congregations in the provision of social services and introduced an innovative new course on social work and religion. Dr. Cnaan has published numerous articles in scientific journals on a variety of social issues. He is the co-author of *The Newer Deal: Social Work and Religion in Partnership, The Invisible Caring Hand: American Congregations and the Provision of Welfare*, and *The Other Philadelphia Story: How Local Congregations Support Quality of Life in Urban America*. Currently, along with Carl Milofsky from Bucknell University, Dr. Cnaan edits the *Handbook of Community Movements and Local Organizations*.

SECTION I

CONCEPTUAL ANALYSIS

Introduction

Ram A. Cnaan
Stephanie C. Boddie

The first section of this volume focuses on setting the conceptual and methodological background for the study of the efficacy of faith-based social services. Given that social science has largely neglected the study of religious issues for more than half a century, and because of the complexity of the new faith-based initiative as outlined in the following Chapter 1, by Cnaan and Boddie, we must set the foundation that will help us form a benchmark for acceptable standards and procedures for such future study. In this section, we ask a set of scholars to answer one set of questions: What are the challenges and methods that will enable us to assess the efficacy of faith-based social services? The responses are quite varied, and combined they form a beginning understanding of the challenges that lie ahead.

McGrew and Cnaan (Chapter 2) open our volume by discussing how social science research neglected the world of religion and religious-based services for almost a century. This neglect resulted in the current immaturity of the field, which lacks methodological tools and consistent conceptual language for studying faith-based service providers. Using the Philadelphia Census of Congregations (PCC), they illustrate problems such as lack of shared language and definitions by academicians and the faith community, and lack of basic knowledge such as building sampling frames. They show how the PCC dealt with these

[Haworth co-indexing entry note]: "Introduction." Cnaan, Ram A., and Stephanie C. Boddie. Co-published simultaneously in *Journal of Religion & Spirituality in Social Work* (The Haworth Pastoral Press, an imprint of The Haworth Press, Inc.) Vol. 25, No. 3/4, 2006, pp. 3-4; and: *Faith-Based Social Services: Measures, Assessments, and Effectiveness* (ed: Stephanie C. Boddie, and Ram A. Cnaan)

problems, and call for refining the language used by researchers for further study of congregations and their services.

George M. von Furstenberg (Chapter 3), in a comprehensive and insightful conceptual review, invites us to acknowledge the many challenges that are facing research in this area. He notes the problems inherent in comparing these sets of providers and identifying the real causes of outcome differences. He eloquently demonstrates how difficult it is to assess what it is to be a service provider and what the faith-factor means.

In Chapter 4, Bruce A. Thyer laments the neglect or contempt that faith-based social care programs are receiving. Public funds, however, bring about the expectation for public scrutiny. Thyer, along with others in this section, wonders how best to be able to measure the efficacy of faith-based organizations. He suggests the use of conventional empirically-oriented program evaluation research as a means to justify their receipt of ongoing support from public funds. With awareness that negative results may be politically difficult to stomach, Thyer proposes that research findings be scrutinized by the faith-based community to help make tough, empirically-based, decisions on funding priorities.

David A. Zanis and Ram A. Cnaan (Chapter 5) join the other authors in reflecting on how best to tackle the challenge of faith-based social service evaluation. Borrowing from the rich literature on randomized controlled clinical trials (RCCT) they suggest a model of serving people who are in a community drug and alcohol program. Their model trains program staff and then splits the trained staff into two groups: one with secular traditional services and the other with the exact same services plus a religious component. Clients are assigned to each such site randomly.

Finally, Robert L. Fischer and Judson D. Stelter (Chapter 6) first review the scope of faith-based social services and then describe promising avenues for enhancing the current understanding of outcomes of FBO services such as (1) adopting outcome measurement practices in use within the current nonprofit sector, and (2) developing more rigorous research designs tailored to the special contexts of faith-based services. Using an agreed-upon set of methods and benchmarks may make the results more acceptable and less contentious.

Chapter 1

Setting the Context:
Assessing the Effectiveness
of Faith-Based Social Services

Ram A. Cnaan
Stephanie C. Boddie

SUMMARY. This paper provides an overview of assessing the effectiveness of newly legislated social policies. In an era of growing public reliance on faith-based social services, it is imperative to be accountable and assess the efficacy and effectiveness of this set of providers. It discusses the paucity of such attempts and the complications involved in measuring effectiveness of social programs, especially when religion is involved. It then reviews the contributions provided in this volume and draws conclusions for future studies. doi:10.1300/J377v25n03_02 *[Article copies available for a fee from The Haworth Document Delivery Service: 1-800-HAWORTH. E-mail address: <docdelivery@haworthpress.com> Website: <http://www.HaworthPress.com> © 2006 by The Haworth Press, Inc. All rights reserved.]*

Ram A. Cnaan, PhD, is affiliated with The School of Social Policy & Practice, University of Pennsylvania.

Stephanie C. Boddie, PhD, is affiliated with George Warren Brown School of Social Work, Washington University in St. Louis.

Address correspondence to: Stephanie C. Boddie, George Warren Brown School of Social Work, One Brookings Drive, Campus Box 1196, St. Louis, MO 63130.

[Haworth co-indexing entry note]: "Setting The Context: Assessing the Effectiveness of Faith-Based Social Services." Cnaan, Ram A., and Stephanie C. Boddie. Co-published simultaneously in *Journal of Religion & Spirituality in Social Work* (The Haworth Pastoral Press, an imprint of The Haworth Press, Inc.) Vol. 25, No. 3/4, 2006, pp. 5-18; and: *Faith-Based Social Services: Measures, Assessments, and Effectiveness* (ed: Stephanie C. Boddie, and Ram A. Cnaan) The Haworth Pastoral Press, an imprint of The Haworth Press, Inc., 2006, pp. 5-18. Single or multiple copies of this article are available for a fee from The Haworth Document Delivery Service [1-800-HAWORTH, 9:00 a.m. - 5:00 p.m. (EST). E-mail address: docdelivery@haworthpress.com].

KEYWORDS. Faith-based service, program effectiveness, faith-based initiatives, evaluation, charitable choice

In the past decade, the balance between the state and faith-based social providers has shifted dramatically. Prior to 1996, faith-based social services, many of which were prominent in the public social service delivery arena, were, in fact, secular in nature. While they contained religious titles such as "Catholic Charities," "Jewish Children and Family Services" or "Episcopal Social Services," they did not preach or disseminate their religious doctrines, hired professionally trained staff who were not necessarily from their own faith tradition, did not celebrate religious holidays with clients, and mirrored their secular counterparts. All of this, however, began to change in 1996.

The Personal Responsibility and Work Opportunity Reconciliation Act of 1996 (P.L. 104-193) contains a special section that has transformed the relationship between the public sector and faith-based social providers. This is section 104 of the Act, also commonly referred to as "Charitable Choice." This provision significantly changes the historic relationship of the religious community and the public sector by opening the door for mixing religion and publicly-supported social services. Charitable Choice outlines the primary feature of this provision as follows:

> The purpose of this section is to allow States to contract with religious organizations, or to allow religious organizations to accept certificates, vouchers, or other forms of disbursement . . . on the same basis as any other non-governmental provider without impairing the religious character of such organizations, and without diminishing the religious freedom of beneficiaries of assistance funded under such program.

The objectives of Charitable Choice are to: (1) encourage states and counties to increase the participation of nonprofit organizations in the provision of federally-funded welfare programs, with specific mention of religious-based organizations; (2) establish eligibility for religious-based organizations as contractors for service on the same basis as other organizations; (3) protect the religious character and employment exemption status of participating religious-based organizations; and (4) safeguard the religious freedom of participants.

Since the enactment of Charitable Choice as part of welfare reform in 1996, the relationship between government and faith-based service providers has undergone a revolution. Congress, the U.S. Supreme Court, and certainly the Bush administration are more receptive to the idea that government can purchase services from faith-based providers, so long as taxpayers are not paying for purely religious services such as the purchase of Bibles, Sunday School materials or clergy salary. This change in the balance between the state and faith-based providers was also transferred to the state level. By 2005, 27 states had enacted legislation with references to faith-based organizations, and 63 percent of states now have an individual or office to serve as a liaison.

A report by the White House Office of Faith-Based and Community Initiatives (2006) revealed that in fiscal year 2005, 10.9% of competitive funds distributed by the seven departments where faith-based offices are in place were directed to faith-based providers. This amounted to an annual increase of seven percent in dollar value and 22 percent increase in the number of awardees who were considered faith-based. In other words, the practice of faith-based social services provision seems to be common and is not showing any signs of phasing out. The interlinking of government and faith-based social service providers was intensified post-Hurricane Katrina. While public services from the city to federal levels failed to prevent the crisis and failed to assist the disaster victims, the only groups that came out shining and revered were the community faith-based organizations (White House, 2006). The government report on the Katrina disaster and post-Katrina response praised the faith-based community, from small churches to the larger organizations, and called upon the public authorities to better integrate them into their systems of care for future events. Again, the role of faith-based social service providers in our public social service system is still on the rise.

As new kids on the block, Charitable Choice and the faith-based initiatives must legitimize the basis for their inclusion in the already-rich tapestry of public social service providers. Their origin was in the 1980s with the anti-big-government sentiment and the rise of the new-federalism camp. While there are many notable examples, we will highlight two that are linked to our topic of assessing efficacy. First, U.S. Senator Dan Coats (R-IN) often told the story of the Union Gospel Mission, a drug-treatment center for homeless men not far from the nation's capital. According to Coats, the mission, under the leadership of John Woods, successfully rehabilitates two thirds of its clients. Just three blocks away is a government-operated shelter with similar goals. Although the government-operated shelter spends 20 times more dollars per person, it boasts only a 10 percent success rate. Senator Coats has an explanation for the disparity: "The Gospel Mission succeeds because it provides more than a meal, more than a drug treatment. It is in the business of spreading the grace of God" (Frame, 1995: 65). Careful social scientists easily refute these high rates of success, but Coats' message is clear: faith-based social services are superior. It is more likely that the Gospel Mission picks and chooses its clients, or the clients self-select, therefore increasing the chance for success. This practice is known as "creaming." The government shelter, on the other hand, does not have this luxury. They are mandated to admit any applicant as long as space is available and no screening is allowed. Comparing the success of a program that creams clients to one that serves any client in need, might make for good politics, but not necessarily for good social science. In addition, the study data come from different sources (as there has not been a single-study comparing both religious and public programs), therefore it is likely that the definitions of success applied are different and would thus contribute to the disparity in reported outcomes.

Second, President Ronald Reagan, who championed new federalism, was the one to plant the seed about the high expectations from faith-based social providers. Reagan reinforced the conservative viewpoint that personal character flaws and government-operated social programs were to blame for poverty:

> The story of the Good Samaritan has always illustrated to me what God's challenge really is. He crossed the road, knelt down, bound up the wounds of the beaten traveler, the pilgrim and carried him to the nearest town. He didn't go running into town and look for a caseworker to tell him that there was a fellow out there that needed help. He took it upon himself. (Denton, 1982, Reagan Home Page, 1997)

It is important to recognize here that policies and the programs they engender reflect the values of those shaping the policy. Reagan had created a new public devil–"the government bureaucrat"–by pitting the godless, uncaring, bureaucratic caseworker against the Good Samaritan. As part of his campaign against the power of professionals and civil servants, he relied on faith-based providers to be part of the picture by painting them as flawless angels.

The ideological campaign was fruitful. In less then two decades, Charitable Choice was enacted, the White House office of Faith-based and Community Initiatives was formed, faith-based offices were established in seven key federal departments, and more and more grants have been given to faith-based providers. In many ways this is a paradigm shift and all indications are that this practice is here to stay. What we lack, however, is rigorous empirical knowledge about the efficacy of these social service providers. As McGrew and Cnaan demonstrate in the following chapter, years of academic neglect and avoidance of studying religious-related topics have left social scientists of our time lacking the know-how and the real experience in studying faith-based organizations. Many concepts are not well defined, credibility of many methods is doubtful, and years of research are sorely missing.

Furthermore, the faith-based initiative proponents have set the bar so high that no other social service agencies could possibly meet their unrealistic expectations. No social service agency that deals with unemployed people, substance abusers, or homeless people can claim an eighty percent rate of success and be taken seriously. It is without question that Senator Coats' numbers are very inflated and do not represent a real and fair comparison. But our lack of knowledge is even more embarrassing. We do not know if faith-based social services are at all effective, and when compared to secular (private, public or nonprofit) social services, if they are performing equally, better or worse. In this volume, we set out focus on answering this question.

HOW DO WE KNOW?

The question of "how do we know?" has puzzled people for many generations. This epistemological search to understand and control events started at the dawn of civilization, but accelerated in the enlightenment era. The idea of science is that internal, intuitive, a-priori knowledge is subjective and often misleading. Such knowledge is often based on ideology or personal wish, and is akin to belief rather than true knowledge. Accordingly, only a-posteriori, external, and empirical knowledge should be considered relevant knowledge for policy making. This is knowledge that is objective and originates through systematic empirical study.

Whenever a new mode of intervention is proposed or a new public policy is set, scholars and politicians alike argue its merits. Whether its focus is seat-belt use in cars or the long-term benefits of Head-Start programs, the debate often centers on the question, "how do we know that the policy really works?" Put differently, how do we know that tax-payer money is put to good use? In almost all public policy issues, ideology and beliefs drive a large share of the rhetoric. Without conviction and an army of believers, no policy or societal change would be legislated and accepted. But in areas where there has been little empirical study, the debate and legislation is founded almost entirely on a-priori convictions. Often there is insufficient time, money, and partial interests to scientifically investigate the proposed changes before they are enacted, but once new policies are approved they must be followed with rigorous and impartial studies. Similarly, those supporting and those opposing a certain policy are threatened by the possible findings from an empirical investigation and prefer to stay with their own a-priori knowledge/beliefs rather than be faced with risky findings.

Real social science is predicated on the principle of "rule of evidence." In the legal field, the rule of evidence is a key principle whereby any alleged matter of fact that is submitted for investigation at a judicial trial is either established or disproved. Put differently, while expert witnesses of opposing sides claim to the validity of opposing realities, the task of the judge is to determine whether a claim is supported or not based on the evidence presented. The same ought to apply in public policy. The ideological debate and personal knowledge can only go so far. At a certain point, the rule of evidence must apply, and opponents and supporters must rely on careful studies which provide replicable results using standardized methods. This rule calls upon researchers to conduct studies as bias-free as possible, and provide valid and reliable scientific evidence that cannot be refuted.

When Charitable Choice was passed, involving religion as it did, it engendered an even higher level of ideology and a-priori conviction in the public debate than usual. While President Clinton was a strong supporter of faith-based social services, they are more commonly associated with President George W. Bush, who established The White House Office of Faith-Based and Community Initiatives in 2001. Opponents and proponents alike use much rhetoric and can hardly substantiate their claims with solid empirical knowledge. When claims are made in political speeches that a faith-based homeless shelter or a faith-based drug and alcohol rehabilitation center is ten times more efficient than their secular counterparts, or alternatively that faith-based organizations see service provision as merely an opportunity to proselytize, those claims are typically based on pure a-priori beliefs or, at best, a few carefully chosen case studies. In this debate, the ideological fight over the role of religion in civil life conflates the discussion and makes the sides more argumentative and fearful of real empirical results.

It seems likely that Charitable Choice won political support at least in part due to the high level of trust Americans have in faith-based organizations. For example, when residents of Maryland were asked in 1999 to rate organizations according to how well they do "the job you expect," places of worship, such as churches, synagogues or mosques were ranked first with a mean of 8.0 (on a scale of ten). A replication of the same survey two years later, in 2001, showed that places of worship retained their top rank, with the rising to 8.5 (Maryland Association of Nonprofit Organizations, 2002). Similarly, the Pew Research Center for the Public & The Press (2000) reported that the majority of Americans support using public funds for social services provided through congregations and other faith-based organizations. Trust and widespread support are important politically and do serve as indirect evidence that faith-based social services are generally helpful, but this kind of evidence is no substitute for formal, rigorous studies of the efficacy and efficiency of those services. After all, public attitude may be based on political marketing and may be wrong.

As often is the case in public policy, without rigorous data and with full conviction, on January 29, 2001 President George W. Bush called for a new era of partnership between the government and religious groups. Proponents hailed the faith-based initiative. On that same day, CNN's Tucker Carlson on The Spin Room declared that: "Study after study shows these faith-based initiatives work better, much better in most cases, than government ones." Similarly, William Donahue, president of the Catholic League for Religious and Civil Rights, told The Washington Times, "Faith-based initiatives not only work better than their secular counterparts, they do so at a fraction of the cost" (Peres, 2001).

Proponents of the faith-based initiative claimed that faith-based services are superior to the secular services as they can use committed volunteers, available resources, spirit of care, have a holistic perspective, instill a spirit of hope, and are helping workers and clients to fulfill a higher goal (Carlson-Thies & Skillen, 1996; Sherman, 1999). The promise was even greater for the Black community, as it suffers from greater social needs and discrimination, and as rates of religiosity and the role of the organized church are more prominent in the Black community (Alex-Assensoh, 2004; DiIulio, 1999). Surprisingly, in the political debate over faith-based social service provision, the opponents of this initiative rarely counter this unrealistic expectation of efficacy superiority. Most arguments against the faith-based initiative have centered on the separation of church and state, rights of clients, and protection of service employees. The myth about the high efficacy of faith-based social services was not challenged and was assumed to be true. But, like in a Greek tragedy, it also trapped faith-based social service providers, as they are now expected to demonstrate a high-level of performance that is in fact barely short of impossible.

A more realistic expectation comes from the field of contract theory. Put simply, everything being equal, the greater the number of providers bidding on a contract, the higher the likelihood that the contract will be carried out to the satisfaction of the contracting agency and at a lower price. The idea is that when a group of providers bid for service, the quality of work will be more-or-less equal but the cheaper bid will save money. Thus, faith-based social providers enlarge the pool of potential bidders, lowering the cost of public social services.

Similarly, and a little less publicly, social scientists, who have a responsibility to paint an objective picture, have been asking themselves "Are faith-based social service providers really that much better or even better at all? If they can in fact provide services equal to or better than secular alternatives, can they really do it more cost-effectively? How can we find out?" In 1996, and even by 2001, there was almost no solid empirical data to examine. This volume represents a slice of the first major wave of research on the effectiveness of faith-based services, but there is still far too little reliable information to properly answer those questions.

THIS VOLUME'S MISSION AND BOUNDARIES

In this volume, we set forth to tackle the essential questions of whether faith-based social services work effectively and efficiently compared to secular alternatives, but we give equal focus to methodological concerns which must be addressed along the way to answering that question. However, before we turn our attention on this question, it is worth taking a moment to explain what is *not* included in this discussion.

First, we are not concerned here with specifically religious or spiritual interventions. There are many religious practices that are and will no doubt continue to be advocated as good social interventions. For example, there is a growing body of literature on the health or mental-health efficacy of meditation, intercessory prayer, and forgiveness education. Some clinical trials or controlled studies have been carried out to assess the efficacy of these modalities in health and social interventions (Freedman & Enright, 1996; Matthews, Marlowe, & MacNutt 2000; Targ & Levine, 2002). The difference between these studies and those we focus on in this volume is that these studies focus on the religious character of *interventions* whereas we focus on the religious character of *organizations*.

One example of a religious intervention that utilizes religion as part of the service provided to the client is Rational Emotive Spiritual Therapy (REST). The integration of a cognitive behavioral therapy approach called Rational Emotive Therapy (RET) with a spiritual or faith-based component–is cited in the literature as promising (Ellis, 2000; Hatcher & McGuire, 2001). In the REST model, the spiritual component is fully integrated into all aspects of the cognitive-behavioral intervention. The literature suggests that both the cognitive-behavioral and faith-based aspects of this intervention, which focuses on emotional healing, has the potential to reduce criminal recidivism, as well as improve problem-solving skills and psychological well-being (O'Connor, 2002).

Section 104 of PRWORA did not specify methods of intervention, but rather encouraged public funds to be used in contracting with faith-based organizations. These organizations can use religious interventions (if they are not perceived as proselytizing) or secular interventions, but are distinct from other agencies that are also contracted by the state. The key difference is in their organizational character: they are faith-based organizations. While not all faith-based organizations are alike, differing in organizational structure and the role religion plays in them (Jeavons, 1998; Smith & Sosin, 2001; Unruh & Sider, 2001), they are the set of organizations that is the focus of the faith-based initiative. Thus, we are not focusing on religious or spiritual interventions per se, but, rather on the efficacy of one group of organizations that is religiously affiliated versus another group of organizations that is secular in nature.

Second, we do not focus here on whether and how the personal religion of social service recipients affects the outcome of certain interventions. This question has also been studied, and will certainly continue to be studied (Tonigan, Miller, & Schermer, 2002). Whether, and how, religious beliefs and practices of social workers and other service workers affect social service delivery are important questions, but our scope here is limited to the nature of the serving organizations. This limited scope closely matches the recent policy initiative: even under PRWORA, religious organizations are not allowed to use public funds for any overtly religious practices, nor are they allowed to impose any standards of religious beliefs or practices on recipients of publicly funded services. Yet, many of the proponents of the faith-based initiative are basing their expectations on the religiosity of the workers and their commitment to God as motivating them to be especially attuned to clients' needs.

What we are concerned with in this volume is the efficacy of certain service organizations versus other service organizations regardless of the interventions applied by specific workers, regardless of the workers' own beliefs, and regardless of the manner in which these beliefs are actualized by the workers (see discussion by von Furstenberg in this volume). Put differently, although there is ample evidence to indicate that religion can have a positive impact on individuals' wellbeing, and that workers who are motivated by religious beliefs may be more committed to their clients, no such knowledge exists regarding regular social services that are provided by faith-based organizations.

Efficacy studies are always very difficult to implement, but efficacy studies of faith-based social service providers encounter some unique obstacles which render them particularly troublesome. To use a metaphor, in this volume we do not ask if "holy water" is better than "regular water" in alleviating thirst. What we do ask is if water given by holy hands is superior to water given by secular hands in alleviating thirst. If the source of the water (funding) is the same, do the holy (religious) hands somehow make a difference in the alleviation of thirst (efficacy of care) because it is better under the sacred auspices? Clearly, when social and personal services are concerned, the complexity of the "water" intensifies. The process or relationships between a worker and client may have as high an impact as the prescribed intervention. So, one may ask: "If faith-based services are proven more effective–is it because they have more devoted workers or is because they are having the religious hallow around them?"

It is difficult to establish a comparison with secular service providers for several reasons. Since faith-based organizations tend to have different (and more varied) organizational structures from their secular counterparts, even comparable groups are tricky to identify. The fact that two organizations provide the same service does not guarantee that their budgets, personnel, policies, experiences, workers' morale, technical know-how, and buildings are of the same nature-all of which can be intervening variables in assessing efficacy. The organizational literature suggests that large and experienced organizations with professional staff are, on average, better at serving poor people. However, such organizations can come from either the faith-based or secular set of social service providers. In fact, some of the contributions to this volume will explore the possibility that observed differences in outcomes may be the result of organizational characteristics that are not faith-related.

Even if organizational variables can be equalized, there remains a possible selection bias. Can clients be forced to go to a religious service provider? It would be clearly unethical. Charitable Choice specifically guarantees clients of a choice to bail out of a religious service provider if they wish. It is thus very difficult to resolve the question of whether a difference in outcomes is due to a difference in the quality of service, or due to a difference in the kinds of people who seek out faith-based providers.

Another major hurdle in evaluation has been the need to account for the inconsistent information flow about Charitable Choice. We are following a new policy that has been implemented at various paces in various states and cities. Even within the same community, not all actors are informed and understand the new policy in a uniform manner. For example, Stanziola and Schmitz (2003) studied the implementation of contracting with faith-based day-care providers in Lee County, Florida. They concluded that "any devolutionary policy that aims to aggressively include faith-based organizations in the provision of social services will face the challenge of weak information flow mechanisms within the industry." Not the least of these problems of implementation is the lack of knowledge and occasional opposition of the public officials who are in charge of contracting or supervising the work of the faith-based social service providers. As the White House (2001) noted, "there exists a widespread bias against faith and community-based organizations in Federal social service programs" (p. 3). Charitable Choice has been almost entirely ignored by Federal administrators, who have done little to help, and have not required state and local governments to comply with the new rules for involving faith-based providers.

These and other challenges have made the first wave of rigorous study both conceptually and logistically difficult. Compounded by politicians' and policy makers' reluctance to seek answers beyond their own ideologies, our scientific knowledge as to the efficacy of faith-based social services is indeed limited.

The purpose of this volume is to collect some of the wisdom and experiences a group of top scholars and leaders in the field have collected so far. We approached scholars who are experts in research methods and asked them to reflect on the challenges facing empirical researchers, and we approached scholars who have "gotten their hands dirty" and could share from their real-life experience. This volume is therefore divided into two main sections: conceptual/methodological contributions and empirical contributions. As expected, most contributions raise more questions than answers. Yet, we are convinced this volume will advance the field of assessing faith-based social services, and some rudimentary questions will accordingly be resolved and replaced with more sophisticated ones. Many terminological questions regarding faith-based social services are at last reaching some clarity, and the field is coming to consensus on what the important questions are. Furthermore, growing awareness of the common intervening variables will guide the work of future researchers as they design studies which account for them.

CONCLUSIONS

Any field of study that has been neglected for such a long time must be treaded in as carefully as a completely unknown field. One cannot move ahead at full speed and apply existing methods before carefully assessing their relevance. This is especially the case with assessing the effectiveness of organizations in a field as contentious as the role of religion in public life. The ideological and political stakes are so high that no single study or single method can persuade believers to change their views. To achieve this, we need a large set of rigorous studies employing various research designs and methods focusing on various subsets of industries (such as welfare to work, drug and alcohol rehabilitation, child day care, and adult education) in which faith-based providers play a key role.

One issue that must be acknowledged in assessing the effectiveness of faith-based social services is their potential replication. The more an intervention is religion-specific, the less likely it is that other faith traditions will adopt it. Thus, evaluation of faith-based social services must precisely report the amount of religiosity in the program and its specificity to one or more faith traditions.

This volume sets the foundation for such an endeavor. The first part of the volume addresses conceptual and methodological challenges involved in the study of faith-based social services and offers a variety of possible solutions. The latter part reports on a few select studies that have attempted to empirically answer the effectiveness question. The findings are tentative and may signify the end of the first wave of studies. They suggest that faith-based social services are neither superior nor inferior to secular services, yet clients report liking them. But even this generalization needs replication from other studies before it can be accepted as conclusive. Without serious commitment to evaluation research that will rigorously assess the effectiveness of faith-based social services, practitioners and policy-makers will continue to rely on a-priori knowledge that is based on pre-conceived ideas and ideology without scientific evidence.

REFERENCES

Alex-Assensoh, Y. M. (2004). Taking the sanctuary to the streets: Race and community development in Columbus, Ohio. *The Annals of the American Academy of Political and Social Science,594*, 79-91.

Carlson-Thies, S. W., & Skillen, J. W. (1996). *Welfare in America: Christian perspectives on a policy in crisis.* Grand Rapids, MI: Eerdmans Publishing Company.

Cnaan, R. A., with Boddie, S. C., Handy, F., Yancey, G., & Schneider, R. (2002). *The invisible caring hand: American congregations and the provision of welfare.* New York: New York University Press.

Denton, H. H. (1982, April, 14). Reagan urges more church aid for needy. *Washington Post,* p. A3.

DiIulio, J. J. Jr. (1999). Black churches and the inner-city poor. In: C. H. Foreman Jr. (Ed.), *The African American* predicament (pp. 116-140). Washington, DC: Brookings Institution.

Ellis, A. (2000). Can rational emotive behavior therapy be effectively used with people who have devout beliefs in God and religion? *Professional Psychology, Research and Practice, 3*, 29-33.

Frame, R. (1995). Religious nonprofits fight for government funds. *Christian Century, 39*, 14, 65.

Freedman, S. R., & Enright, R. D. (1996). Forgiveness as an intervention goal with incest survivors. *Journal of Consulting and Clinical Psychology, 64*, 983-992.

Goggin, M., & Orth, D. (2001). *How faith-based and secular organizations tackle housing for the homeless.* Albany, NY: Roundtable on Religion and Social Welfare Policy, Nelson A. Rockefeller Institute of Government.

Hatcher, R., & McGuire, J. (2001). Offense-focused problem solving: Preliminary evaluation of a cognitive skills program. *Criminal Justice Behavior, 28*, 564-567.

Jeavons, T. (1998). Identifying characteristics of "religious" organizations: An exploratory proposal. In N. J. Demerath III, P. D. Hall, T. Schmitt, & R. H.Williams (Eds.), *Sacred companies: Organizational aspects of religion and religious aspects of organizations* (pp. 79-96). New York, NY: Oxford University Press.

Maryland Association of Nonprofit Organizations (2002). *Protecting the trust: Revisiting public attitudes about charities in Maryland.* Baltimore: Author. Retrieved, December 2, 2005 from: http://www.marylandnonprofits.org/html/explore/documents/public_trust.pdf

Matthews, M. E., Marlowe, S. M., & MacNutt, F. S. (2000). Effects of intercessory prayer on patients with rheumatoid arthritis. *Southern Medical Journal, 93*, 1178-1187.

O'Connor, T. P. (2002). Introduction: Religion-offenders-rehabilitation: Questioning the relationship. *Journal of Offender Rehabilitation, 35*, 1-10.

Peres, E. (April 9, 2001). Lead us not into temptation. *The American Prospect.* Retrieved December 2, 2005 from: http://www.prospect.org/web/page.ww?section=root&name=ViewPrint&articleId=5711

The Personal Responsibility and Work Opportunity Reconciliation Act of 1996, H.R. 3734, 104th Congress, 2nd Session, P.L. 104-193.

Pew Research Center for the Public & The Press (2000). *Religion and politics: The ambivalent majority.* Washington, DC: Author. Retrieved December 2, 2005 from: http://people-press.org/reports/display.php3?ReportID=32

The Reagan Home Page (1997, August version) *Reagan's Speech to the Annual Prayer Breakfast.* Retrieved December 2nd, 2005 from: http://pages.prodigy.com/christianhmsc/speech1.htm

Sherman, A. (June, 1999). Faith-based approaches to social services: Lessons learned. Hudson Institute. Retrieved June 1st, 2005 from: http://www.hudson.org/index.cfm?fuseaction=publication_details&id=112

Smith, S. R., & Sosin, M. R. (2001). The varieties of faith-related agencies. *Public Administration Review, 61*, 651-669.

Stanziola, J., & Schmitz, T. (2003). The Impact of devolution on organizational effectiveness: An exploratory case study of faith-based child care. *The Qualitative Report, 8*, 655-675.

Targ, E. F., & Levine, E. G. (2002). The efficacy of the mind-body-spirit group for women with breast cancer: A randomized controlled trial. *General Hospital Psychiatry, 24*, 238-248.

Tonigan, J. S., Miller, W. R., & Schermer, C. (2002). Atheists, agnostics and Alcoholics Anonymous. *Journal of Studies on Alcohol, 63*, 534-541.

Unruh, H. R., & Sider, R. (2001, November). Religious elements of faith-based social service programs: Types and integrative strategies. Paper presented at the Society for the Scientific Study of Religion Annual Meeting, Columbus, OH.

The White House. (2001). *Unlevel playing field: Barriers to participation by faith-based and community organizations in federal social service programs.* Washington, DC: Author. Retrieved December 2, 2005 from: http://www.whitehouse.gov/news/releases/2001/08/20010816-3-report.pdf

The White House. (2006). *The federal response to hurricane Katrina: Lessons learned.* Washington DC: Retrieved March 15, 2006 from: http://www.religionandsocialpolicy.org/docs/press_releases/katrina-lessons-learned.pdf

The White House Office of Faith-Based and Community Initiatives (2006). *Grants to faith-based organizations fiscal year 2005: Based on a review of 130 competitive programs and 28 program areas at seven federal agencies.* Washington, DC: Retrieved March 15, 2006 from: http://www.whitehouse.gov/government/fbci/final_report_2005.pdf

Chapter 2

Finding Congregations:
Developing Conceptual Clarity
in the Study of Faith-Based Social Services

Charlene C. McGrew
Ram A. Cnaan

SUMMARY. The need to assess the effectiveness of faith-based social interventions is pressing. On the one hand, politicians and pundits claim that faith-based organizations are impressively successful and inexpensive. On the other hand, critics claim that faith-based organizations lack the capacity to carry out social services. However, rigorously-collected empirical data is just beginning to appear and is still in short supply, particularly congregations. In this paper, we discuss some critical methodological and conceptual problems that arise from years of academic neglect of faith-based social service provision. We demonstrate how our attempt to create a comprehensive account of congregation-based social services in Philadelphia necessitated defining even such basic terms as

---

Charlene C. McGrew and Ram A. Cnaan are affiliated with the School of Social Policy & Practice, University of Pennsylvania.

Address correspondence to: Charlene C. McGrew, School of Social Policy & Practice, University of Pennsylvania, 3815 Walnut Street, Philadelphia, PA 19104 (E-mail: cmcgrew@ssw.upenn.edu).

[Haworth co-indexing entry note]: "Finding Congregations: Developing Conceptual Clarity in the Study of Faith-Based Social Services." McGrew, Charlene C., and Ram A Cnaan. Co-published simultaneously in *Journal of Religion & Spirituality in Social Work* (The Haworth Pastoral Press, an imprint of The Haworth Press, Inc.) Vol. 25, No. 3/4, 2006, pp. 19-37; and: *Faith-Based Social Services: Measures, Assessments, and Effectiveness* (ed: Stephanie C. Boddie, and Ram A. Cnaan) The Haworth Pastoral Press, an imprint of The Haworth Press, Inc., 2006, pp. 19-37.

"congregation" and devising novel methods for identifying and gathering information from congregations. doi:10.1300/J377v25n03_03

KEYWORDS. Program effectiveness, faith-based interventions, faith-based organizations, faith-based social services

In face of recent public demand for trustworthy information about the scope and effectiveness of religious organizations' work in the social service arena, social work scholars have embarrassingly little to offer. Proponents of faith-based initiatives trumpet the many ways in which faith-based services outshine secular alternatives, offering as evidence case studies which perfectly illustrate their claims. Opponents worry about establishment of religion, unregulated and unethical service provision, and a regression to "pregovernmental" social welfare (Belcher, Fandetti, & Cole, 2004). Meanwhile, scholars, policy-makers, and evidence-based practitioners turn in vain to the professional literature for help sorting out whether and when faith-based service providers are effective, and why.

Empirical studies which have been published in the last few years represent only a start at answering these questions. Jason Scott's (2003) thorough review of research literature on faith-based organizations in social service delivery lists very few studies from before the passage of Charitable Choice in 1996 (see also Cnaan, Wineburg, & Boddie, 1999). Of the studies conducted since, most are exploratory and descriptive; very few directly evaluate effectiveness. For example, a recent study (Monsma & Soper, 2003) which rigorously compared the effectiveness of 17 welfare-to-work programs of five types in Los Angeles is rightly regarded as one of the most important studies to date, despite the very small number of organizations representing each type, simply because so few rigorous studies exist. As Fischer and Stelter (see this volume) point out, the lack of systematic data can be attributed to the youth of the field. But whereas the Charitable-choice legislation dates only to 1996, faith-based organizations have been part of the social provision landscape for centuries. The field is not really new; rather it has lain fallow.

The gap in the knowledge is partly explained by a deep rift between a secular professional field and religious organizations and the related division between government and religious social service providers which characterized most of the twentieth century. The recent rush to fill the gap has highlighted a number of methodological issues that must be addressed as we seek to give valid empirical answers to the questions critically important for policy and practice. Because the field is underdeveloped, it suffers from a lack of consistency in definitions of basic terms and a lack of collective experience in identifying and gathering information from the major participants.

The information gap is deep and wide (Johnson, 2002). The last series of comprehensive works on congregations were carried out by Paul H. Douglas (1926) who studied congregations (mostly Presbyterians) until the 1950s. We need to know what organizations exist, what they do, how and why they do it, and what effects they have. This paper focuses on several conceptual and methodological issues involved in answering those questions. After illustrating the current lack of conceptual clarity in the field, we show how one of the present authors' large research projects set out to answer some relatively straightforward questions and found it was necessary to create definitions of key terms and devise new approaches to finding religious congregations along the way. The questions were, what is the scope of congregation-based social service provision in Philadelphia, and what is its approximate replacement value? At the outset of the study, there was no existing social-science based definition of a religious congregation, and no list of local congregations which was remotely comprehensive.

WHY THE GAP?

Social science scholars' lack of attention to religious organizations no doubt has many causes, but it seems that there are at least two major wedges driven between the field and faith, at least in the United States. First, the federal government's dramatic broadening of social services under the New Deal at once nationalized, professionalized, and secularized the field. The Welfare State took over many of the functions of Charity. Some religious organizations remained, or became, part of the field by professionalizing and focusing on service provision as their only or essential mission. These organizations include the Red Cross, the Salvation Army, and semi-independent service organizations of major denominations, such at Catholic Charities. Local congregations seemed to have disappeared from the social sciences radar screen by the middle of the twentieth century. In fact they continued to provide emergency financial relief, food, and shelter, and counsel much as they always had, but for the most part their *ad hoc* and unofficial services were marginalized by scholars as therefore inconsequential and irrelevant. We are now beginning to see that those services, patchwork though they are, comprise a much bigger piece of the social welfare quilt than has been previously acknowledged.

The second wedge comes with the "science" of "social science." The rigorous, empirically driven methodology of science seems awkward, and not infrequently unwelcome, in the study of religious matters, dominated as they are by received authority, personal reflection, and normative teaching. Although among sociologists there is a long tradition of studying religion, social scientists of the latter half of the century were for the most part content to ignore religion almost entirely (Wuthnow, 2004). And there is bad blood between religion and science; we are forever reminded of Galileo recanting under the Inquisition. The power structure has been reversed. In the academy, at least, science has triumphed as the tool for uncovering truth, but despite predictions to the contrary (e.g., Berger, 1967). The population of the U.S., among the most technologically and scientifically advanced societies in the world, remains stubbornly religious in the 20th century (Finke & Stark, 1992; Gallup & Lindsay, 1999; Roof, 1993). In their quest to be recognized as research scientists and professionals in practice, social workers and social work scholars tend to ally with secular worldviews and need-based (as opposed to church membership-based) service provision (Cnaan, Wineburg, & Boddie, 1999).

Evidence-based practice seems, at least to secular practitioners, the very antithesis of faith-based practice. Given an empirical study which indicates that intervention "A" is more effective than intervention "B," a practitioner committed to evidence based practice would, other things being equal, recommend method A over method B (Gibbs & Gambrill, 2002). However, given an empirical study which suggests that memorizing the Qur'an speeds recovery from drug addiction, it seems quite unlikely that a Baptist church-based rehabilitation program would adopt the practice. Hence, success of one religious treatment may be inapplicable to other religious traditions.

In fact, many a conservative Baptist pastor would confirm openly the social worker's suspicion that his church uses whatever social services it provides as a platform for Christian evangelism. What clergy might perceive as an attempt to go beyond temporal, physical needs to meet eternal spiritual needs is likely to be seen by secular professionals as outright unethical proselytism. Religious-based services may also be perceived as amateurish, especially as services like counseling, one of the commonest congregational services, become increasingly professionalized (Wuthnow, 1990).

So for many reasons the gap in the professional knowledge is not surprising. Yet there is growing consensus among academics and practitioners alike that it is high time to bring all our data-gathering tools into action here. The consensus is again doubly driven. For one thing, the Clinton and George W. Bush administrations brought faith-based service provision back into the center of the public square. Under the Charitable Choice provision of the Personal Responsibility and Work Opportunity Reconciliation Act of 1996, faith-based organizations can compete for public funding on equal footing with secular providers without giving up their essential religious character. Public interest demands that public funding come with accountability, hence new attention on the effectiveness of faith-based services. Like any organizations that seek public support, faith-based organizations and secular service providers alike must demonstrate that their programs are both effective and financially accountable. One group of leaders of diverse stakeholders in the civic sector has charged even public and nongovernmental funders to insist on effective performance and outcome measures from all providers of service which they support (Working Group on Human Needs and Faith-Based and Community Initiatives, 2002).

Another impetus for this area of study is the growing realization that faith-based service provision does not just *potentially* play a large role in the social welfare scene, it *already* plays a large part (Chaves, Konieczny, Beyerlein, & Barman, 1999; Cnaan, Wineburg, & Boddie, 1999; Cnaan, Boddie, Handy, Yancey, & Schneider, 2002; Wuthnow, 1990), and one which is grossly understudied. Below the radar screen congregations provided social services to needy members and nonmembers for many years. In Philadelphia alone, the estimated replacement value of services provided by congregations is about 250 million dollars annually. This piece of data, simply stated, was not so simply come by. The process which enabled us to find this and a vast array of other data about Philadelphia congregations illustrates the conceptual and methodological challenges involved in doing empirical research in a relatively new field, particularly research focus on congregations.

CONCEPTUAL CLARITY

As we scramble to fill the gap, our first order of business as social scientists is to come to some agreement on what we mean by what we say. One legacy of the lack of study of religious social service providers is that we inherit loaded and imprecise religious and political language. Reynolds (1971) pointed out that a concept does not help scientists organize, explain, predict, or understand the world unless they clearly agree on the meaning of that concept. In fact, his definition of conceptual clarity is precisely the degree of agreement between users of a concept on its meaning. Still following Reynolds, there are two kinds of concepts to clarify: those that refer to objects or phenomena, and those that describe qualities of those objects or phenomena. For the present discussion, we desperately need both: terms that consistently label the various kinds of religion-based organizations, and terms the consistently describe their features.

Clarity is just what we lack in discussions of faith-based organizations at the moment. It has been argued that the distinction between faith-based organizations and their secular counterparts is relatively simple, and that the taxonomic challenge is mainly in distinguishing types of faith-based organizations (see Fischer & Stelter in this volume). This statement accurately reflects the sense that most of the conceptual work being done focuses on clarifying the 'faith' element in faith-based programs (Jeavons, 2004; Scott, 2003; Unruh & Sider, 2005), but the first part of the claim is somewhat over-optimistic. The term "faith-based organizations" came into common use at least as much because of what it does not say as what it does. It avoids the use of 'religion' and 'church,' and in fact the need for the term was largely because the collection of religion-related (but not exactly religious) organizations needed a label (Vidal, 2001; Wuthnow, 2004). Not only do different people still mean different things by the term "faith-based organization," but, to borrow Thomas Jeavons' (2004) phrase (which in turn echoes Ebaugh, Pipes, Chafetz, & Daniels (2003)), even as individual researchers we might not consistently "know [a faith-based organization] when we see one." Smith and Sosin (2001) offer the term 'faith-related' in place of 'faith-based' to capture the fact that many agencies have religious ties with congregations or other religious bodies but do not base all their actions on faith issues, and thus are uncomfortable with the 'faith-based' label. They look at several dimensions of faith-basedness: funding sources, authority, culture, and "religious coupling," a multidimensional description of the degree to which an organization is linked to faith. Ebaugh and her colleagues (2003) also noted the difficulty of knowing exactly what constituted an FBO, and examined organizations' names, logos, mission statements, funding sources, and hiring practices. Additionally, as Chambre (2001) pointed out, the faith-factor of faith-based organizations often changes significantly within an organization over time.

Sider and Unruh (2004) claimed that because there is no clear definition of "faith-based," the term "faith-based organizations" confuses and divides. They give as the first of several problems due to this lack of clarity, "The lack of clear analytical categories hampers comparative research on the effectiveness of service organizations" (p. 110). In their article they present one of the most sophisticated attempts to date at introducing conceptual precision. They distinguish between organizations and programs, place them in a functional typology with seven divisions along a continuum from "faith-permeated" to "secular," and describe typical features in several dimensions. For example, for religious programs they describe the environment, the content, the main form of integration of religious content with other program components, and the expected connection between religious content and desired outcome.

Jeavons (1997), who was the first to make a serious effort towards developing precise conceptual language to describe religious organizations, treats Sider and Unruh's (2004) typology with respect and appreciation, but not quite acceptance. Particularly relevant here, his third critique of Sider and Unruh's framework is that they fail to address what he sees as possibly the most important question of all: where do congregations fit? How does this typology help solve the pressing question of whether congregations can and should receive government funding under the faith-based-organization legislation? (Jeavons, 2004).

Jeavons (2004) is not even sure that congregations count as "faith-based organizations" in the sense of being potential social-service contracting agencies, and argues that in fact they should not. On the other hand, Chaves, author of the 1998 National Congregation Study, seems to assume that congregations are the normative faith-based organizations, and he and Tsitsos find it necessary to remind their readers that there exist other kinds of faith-based organizations: "Religious congregations–churches, synagogues, mosques–constitute only a subset of the faith-based organizations that some envision playing an expanded role in our social welfare system" (Chaves & Tsitsos, 2001).

So there is not even consensus on whether the set of "faith-based organizations" includes the set of "congregations." One might think that the term "congregation" would be clearer, since religious congregations have been a ubiquitous part of American social life since colonial days. But "congregation" had not been precisely defined in the professional literature. Like other researchers in this new area of study (e.g.,

Ammerman, 1997; Chaves, 2004), one of the present authors was compelled to create precise definitions in the course of designing a major study. The Philadelphia Census of Congregations required us to develop careful definitions of "congregation," and "religiously-based social services." We also had to learn how to overcome the frequent problem of informants not understanding "social service" in the way that we meant the term.

PHILADELPHIA CENSUS OF CONGREGATIONS

Though the Philadelphia Census of Congregations (PCC) provides an immense source of empirical data on the nature and practice of congregations (see preliminary results in Cnaan & Boddie, 2001), here we are concerned with the conceptual and methodological contributions which come from its approach to identifying and contacting representatives of the congregations of Philadelphia. The initial task was simple in concept and enormous in execution: find all the congregations in Philadelphia. The first step was a step backwards: to define congregations. The second step led to many steps; in fact it ultimately led to stepping up and down every street and knocking on many doors in Philadelphia.

Defining a Congregation

A review of the literature revealed that there had been no agreed-upon social science-based empirical definition of congregation. Thus to operationalize the term for our study, we had to refine existing definitions, making reference to both technical and non-technical work. Webster's, for example, defines a congregation as a "religious community (that is) an organized body of believers in a particular locality" (Webster's New Collegiate Dictionary, 1973). Wind and Lewis (1994) provided a helpful starting point for us, as it has for others (see, e.g., Chavez, 2004). Their definition, like others that we found (see Cnaan & Boddie, 2001) recognizably described the concept of congregations, but did not distinguish them from other religious bodies and groups. The PCC pushed us to create a definition which could precisely determine whether an organization or a group (especially any religious gathering) was either a congregation, some other kind of religious organization, or none of the above. For example: is a group of prisoners in the local jail who pray daily a congregation? What about the nuns in the nearby monastery? Pilgrims who gather to pray at St. Peter's cathedral? A weekly neighborhood Bible study? All are examples of people who meet to pray or worship at a particular location, but it seems odd to call them congregations. On the other hand, what distinguishes a home church from the neighborhood Bible study? And how important is a consistent location? Isn't an Amish church whose weekly gatherings move from one member's home to another a congregation?

The term "congregation" clearly needed a more precise definition. Such a definition was critical if we were to estimate the number, size, type, and location, not to mention social impact, of congregations in a way that would be replicable and comparable to other studies. The need to define a congregation can be equated to the need to define a "school" or a "political party." The latter two have been the subjects of intense social science study and hence are well defined; one knows exactly what is implied when the term is invoked. This is not the case with a congregation, as many religious gatherings might or might not be considered congregations.

Using seven criteria–four borrowed from Wind and Lewis (1994) and three that we added–we formulated a working definition for a congregation. This definition does not require that a congregation adhere to a monotheistic faith tradition. It is, therefore, applicable to Hindu and Buddhist traditions as well as to pagan and Satanic groups. The following seven criteria were used:

1. A cohesive group of people with a shared identity, which
2. Meets regularly on an on-going basis;
3. Comes together primarily for worship and has commonly accepted teachings, rituals, and practices;
4. Meets and worships at a designated place;
5. Gathers for worship outside the regular purposes and location of a living or work space;
6. Has an identified religious leader; and
7. Has an official name and some formal structure that conveys its purpose and identity.

This working definition helps to exclude many religious gatherings that are not congregations. Excluded are: groups of people who meet for worship but do so only during certain times of the year, such as college students who occasionally meet during the school year; convents and prison ministries; religious studies groups; social ministries; religious crusades and revivals; shrines and national cathedrals; family devotions; Bible-study groups; regional/national headquarters of religious denominations; yearly meetings; assemblies; religiously-based homeless shelters and hospices; and religious chautauquas. Similarly, group meetings that include religious expressions such as blessings, convocations, and readings of religious texts are not congregations.

No matter what method is used to sample congregations, without a universally accepted definition of congregations, it will be difficult to compare findings across studies. Because different studies may use different definitions, contradictory findings are hard to reconcile as they measure different phenomena. More specificity about what is to be included in the term "congregation" will enable readers to assess the generalizability of the findings.

While the status of congregations as "faith-based organizations" was not of consequence to the PCC, we suggest that congregations should be considered faith-based organizations. When Jeavons (2004) argues that congregations should not be considered faith-based organizations, presumably he has no doubts that congregations are faith-based; what is in doubt is their ability to function as service-providing organizations. As Wuthnow makes clear, the current term "faith-based organization" is essentially an abbreviation of "faith- based service organization." Certainly the argument that a congregation, while faith-based, is not primarily a service organization, has merit. However, for the sake of conceptual clarity, we suggest that congregations be considered a subset of faith-based organizations. This is consistent with most authors' usage (Chavez & Tsistos, 2001; Cnaan, Wineburg, & Boddie, 1999; Scott, 2003; Unruh & Sider, 2005; Vidal, 2001; Wiener, Kirsch, & McCormick, 2002). Furthermore, as the PCC and other studies demonstrate (see, e.g., Ammerman, 2004; Chavez, 1999; Dudley & Roozen, 2001; Saxon-Harrold, Wiener, McCormack, & Weber, 2000; Vidal, 2001; Wuthnow, 2004), congregations play a major part in social service provision even when there are no government contracts involved.

Nevertheless, congregations are a special kind of faith-based organization in terms of their role as social service providers. After all, their primary purpose is not to provide social services, but religious services. Although they contribute a not insignificant portion of formal social services in the United States, their abilities to provide in-depth services are sharply limited (Unruh & Sider, 2005). Our findings (Cnaan et al., 2002) and those of Robert Wuthnow (2004) suggest that congregations' most important role may be in the informal services they provide.

Defining a Congregational Social Service

Before we can assess the effectiveness of congregational-based social service programs, it is essential to define what constitutes a social service in the congregational context. In the PCC, the focus was identifying and categorizing congregation-based social services. This was a tricky proposition. For example, is an AA group that meets on the congregational premises its program? While the congregation provides space and enables the program to exist, the program is only partially its own. If members collect nonperishable food and once every month deliver it to a local homeless shelter, is this a real social service? If 30 members of the congregation regularly assist in a road cleanup that is run by the local authority, is this a congregational social service? Furthermore, if the clergy counsels a child who had an upsetting week at school, is this a social service?

Since church leaders and members do not use the terms "social service" or "social program" consistently, their judgments are not always helpful. When clergy are asked if their congregations offer any social services, they often respond with a "No!" But in further discussion, it becomes clear that what they often mean by the term "social program" or a "social service" is a program sponsored and controlled by the government. Thus, even large-scale day care centers are often not viewed by clergy and congregational representatives as social services, but rather as . . . well, as day care centers. Once again, we see how the linguistic gap between social scientists and representatives of the faith community hinders rigorous studying and understanding of faith-based organizations and programs.

This methodological issue may explain the wide variations in findings between studies that found low and high rates of social services offered by congregations. For example, Chaves (1999) found that only 58% of congregations provide at least one social service, while Silverman (2000) found in the state of California that 100 percent of congregations provide such a service. Unruh and Sider (2005) suggest that such variation in findings probably reflect true variation in social service provision of different samples. Comparing findings from studies in urban contexts, like the PCC, with Chaves' national data, they surmise that congregations in major urban areas demonstrate a higher rate of social service provision than average. This may be true, but given such a small number of studies on which to base such comparisons, it is also quite likely that observed differences can be attributed largely to different working definitions and methodological considerations.

When identifying social services provided by congregations the following questions arise:

1. Does the social service program have to be registered as a separate nonprofit organization with its own 501 (c) (3) designation?
2. Does the service have to be offered on the congregational premises or can it be offered elsewhere (such as cleaning a park or adopting a nursing home)?
3. Must the service have a budget and/or staff to be counted?
4. Does the service have to be on-going, or can a sporadic or seasonal service be counted?
5. Can another organization (such as Boy Scouts of America or AA) use the congregational premises, and if so, should the provision of rent-free meeting space be considered a congregational social service?
6. Can non-members of the congregations be involved in the service provision?
7. Can the service be offered jointly with another congregation, social service organization, or denomination?
8. How can we define a social service in a language that clergy and congregation members will understand? That is the need to speak the language of social ministry which in itself is denominationally specific and not inclusive for social services.

In our work we employed what we saw as the least restrictive reasonable definition: we counted programs as long as they were recognized as programs and not done *ad hoc*. To use the example above, we did not count the clergy who counseled the child as a program, as there is no program with a name and identity, but rather there is a response to an arising need. However, helping in the road cleanup and hosting AA groups are counted as social services in the PCC.

We also learned that most clergy do not recall all the social services that their congregation offers when asked in a general manner. Besides the reluctance to include their congregations' services under the term "social services," the clergy or our key informants frequently could not recall all the services, as some were handled routinely by a sub-committee or group of the congregation and were simply, when asked about, forgotten. To avoid these threats of under-reporting, during the interviews we listed over 200 possible areas of congregational social service and asked the interviewees to recognize which of them were offered by the congregation. Once the interviewee answered positively about a service, we asked if the service was offered formally or only when requested. If offered formally, then we asked where the service was offered, who provided the service, and whether it was offered in cooperation with others. Thus, we minimized the threats of using the wrong terminology and of the interviewees' inability to recall social services.

Sampling Congregations: Mission Possible

Scholars of congregational studies have long noted (Finke & Stark, 1992) that it was impossible to count how many congregations exist in any large city or in the United States as a whole. The problem of counting congregations is due to a few factors. First, there is the problem discussed above, imprecision in the definition of a congregation.

Second, due to the separation of church and state, congregations are exempt from registering with the IRS or any other public authority. As a result, new congregations could come into being and, except for the members of the denomination, or for independent congregations, just the members of the congregation, no one would be aware of them. This contrasts with the European and Canadian policy under which congregations register with the state, and clergy must be graduates of recognized theological seminaries. In many denominations in the United States one's "calling" is often a sufficient ground for becoming a recognized and legitimate clergy person.

Third, congregations, like many other social organizations, have gone through stages of birth, death, and even mergers. For example, in a one-month period in Philadelphia, two new congregations were formed and two others merged into a joint congregation. In other instances, congregations may move to a different neighborhood or change their character to fit the changing environment (Ammerman, 1997).

Fourth, many congregations have such limited trust of the government or secular scholars that they are reluctant to provide any information about themselves. Of all our social institutions, congregations are the most segregated, and often groups of immigrants form their own congregations, opting to remain unknown and free of government intrusion.

Fifth, most attempts to count congregations have been made either by denominations which focused solely on their own congregations or by scholars who have asked denominations to provide their statistics. As a result, small mission congregations, church plants, and/or unpublicized fringe congregations have been consistently overlooked. When we had exhausted all other modes of identifying congregations in Philadelphia, we canvassed the streets in search of congregational signs. This method alone increased our pool of congregations by a remarkable ten percent.

Finally, many congregations are not accessible by phone, do not respond to mailed questionnaires, and operate only a few hours a week. Often the clergy member is the only person who routinely maintains the property, and even he or she works full-time elsewhere, serving as the congregation's leader on weekends and selected times during the week. Identifying such congregations is both time-consuming and costly. Many researchers elect to give up including them in their studies.

In our case, we started with two large lists that were merged together: The City of Philadelphia Property Tax list and the Yellow Pages list of congregations. We assumed that the overwhelming majority of congregations would be listed in these two databases, whose merger would provide the master list for the census. In order to get the rest of the congregations, we took five additional steps. First, we approached every denomination and inter-faith organization in the region and asked each for a list of member congregations. We received fifteen different lists and merged them with our master file. Second, in every interview, the interviewers asked the clergy or key informants to identify congregations with which they collaborated and then asked for their telephone numbers and addresses. We also asked them if they share their space with any other congregation and identify quite a few small and immigrant congregations.

Third, we asked our advisory board and other local congregational leaders to identify missing congregations. Fourth, we collected information from the 2000 census data and from local polling stations. Finally, we undertook walks in the streets of Philadelphia to identify store front churches and other congregations not on our master file.

The original list using Yellow Pages and City Property Tax files included 1,483 congregations in Philadelphia. Of these, 265 were either defunct or did not meet our definition of congregation (for example, there were parsonages, convents, one video store, and private residences of clergy.) Our current database lists 2,120 congregations. In other words, the first-ever congregational census in any American city revealed that the combined Yellow Pages and City Property Tax files correctly identified only 1,218 of the 2,120 known existing congregations (58%). Other master lists such as the National Coalition of Churches or the Glenmary Research Center yielded even lower estimates of congregations in Philadelphia.

GENERALIZABLE RESULTS

The open questions about faith-based organizations are essentially those posed by Chaves and Tsitsos (2001): What do they do? Are they effective? What about them contributes to their unique effectiveness (or lack thereof)? And among the more specific formulations of that last question, what role does the "faith" component play? That is, is their success (or lack thereof) because of, in spite of, or irrelevant to their faith-based nature?

The information collected in the Philadelphia Census of Congregations allows us to generate a wealth of descriptive statistics and examine the correlation between a number of variables. The PCC thus makes a notable empirical contribution. Since we are more concerned with the PCC as an example of refining the precision of definitions and creating a sampling frame, we want to briefly discuss how those aspects of the PCC support general conclusions about faith-based service provision. Much more work is needed in this area, particularly in describing aspects and taxonomic categories of religious organizations. Because the features of social organizations are so varied, in the behavioral and social sciences it is imperative to use multiple trials and comparisons to substantiate a claim for definitive and generalized results (Campbell & Rouso, 1999).

Researchers doing case studies often study big, interesting, unusual, or amenable and convenient congregations, so their results do not generalize to "typical" congregations (Woolever & Bruce, 2002). An ideal sample is a probability sample drawn from an exhaustive sampling frame. So far, in the United States the best sampling frame of congregations in existence is the Philadelphia Census of Congregations described above. However, other cities and towns should also be studied with such intensity to create comprehensive congregational lists. But note its major limitation: strictly speaking, results are only generalizable to Philadelphia. The more different an area is from Philadelphia, the less likely its congregations are to behave like Philadelphia congregations. It is also the case that congregations are formed and dissolved every month, so the list, which took many months to compile, was in some sense outdated before it was even finished.

There are several studies which make a good attempt at being nationally representative samples: the U.S. Congregational Life survey and the National Study of Congregations. These surveys, though, suffer from poor underlying sampling frames–recall that in Philadelphia, only about half the congregations turned up on the obvious sources; it is likely that the national studies had similarly gaping holes in their sampling frames. Here, the generalizability is not limited to a particular region in the U.S. (though it is, of course, limited to the U.S.) But it is limited in the sense that the samples were drawn from easy-to-find congregations and are thus not representative of hard-to-find congregations.

Generalizability of the PCC and other studies of faith-based organizations is also limited by the prevailing lack of conceptual clarity discussed above. Further rigorous studies strengthen findings not just because results can be replicated, but because rigorous studies drive researchers to clarify definitions.

There are, of course, many other challenges both conceptual and methodological. In their recent article on improving the evidence base on faith-based services, Fischer and Stelter (2005) offer suggestions for dealing with selection bias and certain analytical challenges particularly relevant to studying faith-based service provision, and devote significant attention to the development of appropriate and rigorous outcome measures more in line with secular non-profit standards. Saxon-Harrold and colleagues (2000) found that though most congregations do keep records and do some kind of outcomes measurement, a significant minority do not, for reasons of budget and expertise. In another recent work on effectiveness, Campbell and Glunt (see this volume) outline a research strategy focusing on local service delivery networks, highlighting the interplay of government, non-profit, and faith-based services in a community. Such research on effectiveness is crucial in answering the pressing questions, and must be built on a foundation of well-defined concepts and consistent ways of identifying faith-based organizations.

CONCLUSION

We have developed here an account of where research on the most prevalent type of faith-based social services stands and where some of our recent work sits in relation to it. Our focus here has been more on congregations than on non-congregational service providers, because congregational work is where we have the most experience. The differences between those organizations, however, are critical and very much a part of the conceptual clarification which we need. Our experience with the Philadelphia Census of Congregations taught us how undertaking a rigorous empirical study forced the development of conceptual clarity along the way. It is our hope that by outlining lessons learned in that vein and laying out some methodological ideas, we have shown at least a few directions in which further studies can similarly contribute to both conceptual clarity and the body of reliable empirical data in the field of faith-based social service provision.

REFERENCES

Ammerman, N. T. (1997). *Congregations & community.* New Brunswick, NJ: Rutgers University Press.

Ammerman, N. (2004). *Pillars of faith: American congregations and their partners, building faith, building community.* Berekely, CA: University of California Press.

Belcher, J. R., Fandetti, D., & Cole, D. (2004). Is Christian religious conservatism compatible with the liberal social welfare state? *Social Work, 49,* 269-276.

Berger, P. L. (1967). *The sacred canopy: Elements of a sociological theory of religion.* Garden City, NY: Doubleday.

Campbell, D. T., & Rouso M. J. (1999). *Social Experimentation.* Thousand Oaks, CA: Sage.

Chambre, S. M. (2001). The changing nature of "faith" in faith-based organizations: Secularization and ecumenicism in four AIDS organizations in New York City. *Social Service Review, 75,* 435-442.

Chaves, M. (2004). *Congregations in America.* Cambridge, MA: Harvard University Press.

Chaves, M., Konieczny, M. E., Beyerlein, K., & Barman, E. (1999). The National Congregations Study: Background, methods, and selected results. *Journal for the Scientific Study of Religion 38,* 458-476.

Chaves, M., & Tsitsos, W. (2001). Congregations and social services: What they do, how they do it, and with whom. *Nonprofit and Voluntary Sector Quarterly, 30,* 660-683.

Cnaan, R. A., Wineburg, R. J., & Boddie, S. C. (1999). *The newer deal: Social work and religion in partnership.* New York: Columbia University Press.

Cnaan, R. A., & Boddie, S. C. (2001). Philadelphia census of congregations and their social service delivery. *Social Service Review, 75,* 559-580.

Cnaan, R. A., Boddie, S. C., Handy, F., Yancey, G., & Schneider, R. (2002). *The invisible caring hand: American congregations and the provision of welfare.* New York: New York University Press.

Douglass, H. P. (1926). *The church in the changing city.* NY: George Doran.

Dudley, C. S., & A. Roozen, D. A. (2001). *Faith communities today: A report on religion in the United States today.* Hartford, CT: Hartford Institute for Religion Research.

Ebaugh, H. R., Pipes, P. F., Chafetz, J. S., & Daniels, M. (2003). Where's the religion? Distinguishing faith-based from secular social service agencies. *Journal for the Scientific Study of Religion, 42,* 411-426.

Finke, R., & Stark, R. (1992). *The churching of America, 1776-1990: Winners and losers in our religious economy.* New Brunswick, NJ: Rutgers University Press.

Gallup, G. Jr., & Lindsay, D. M. (1999). *Surveying the religious landscape–Trends in U.S. beliefs.* Harrisburg, PA: Morehouse Publishing Company.

Gibbs, L., & Gambrill, E. (2002). Evidence-based practice: Counterarguments to objections. *Research on Social Work Practice, 12,* 452-476.

Jeavons, T. H. (1997). Identifying characteristics of "religious" organizations: An exploratory proposal. In J. Demerath III, P. D. Hall, T. Schmitt, & R. H. Williams (Eds.), *Sacred companies: Organizational aspects of religion and religious aspects of organizations* (pp. 79-95). New York: Oxford University Press.

Jeavons, T. H. (2004). Religious and faith-based organizations: Do we know one when we see one? *Nonprofit and Voluntary Sector Quarterly, 33,* 140-145.

Johnson, B. R. (2002). *Objective hope, assessing the effectiveness of faith-based organizations: A review of the literature.* Philadelphia: Center for Research on Religion and Urban Civil Society (CRRUCS Report), University of Pennsylvania.

Kuhn, T. S. (1962). *The structure of scientific revolutions.* Chicago: University of Chicago Press.

Reynolds, P. D. (1971). *A primer in theory construction.* Boston: Allyn and Bacon.

Roof, W. C. (1993). *A generation of seekers: The spiritual journeys of the baby boom generation.* San Francisco: Harper San Francisco.

Rossi, P. H., & Freeman, H. E. (1993). *Evaluation: A systematic approach (5 Ed.).* Newbury Park, CA: Sage.

Saxon-Harrold, S. K. E., Wiener, S. J., McCormack, M. T., & Weber, M. A. (2001). *America's religious congregations: Measuring their contribution to society.* Washington DC: Independent Sector.

Scott, J. (2003). *The scope and scale of faith-based social services: A review of the research literature focusing on the activities of faith-based organizations in the delivery of social services* (2nd ed.). The Roundtable on Religion and Social Welfare Policy. Retrieved December 12, 2005, from www.religionandsocialpolicy.org/docs/bibliographies/9-4-2002_scope_and_scale.pdf

Sider, R. J., & Unruh, H. R. (2004). Typology of religious characteristics of social service and educational organizations and programs. *Nonprofit and Voluntary Sector Quarterly, 33,* 109-134.

Silverman, C. (2000). *Faith-related communities and welfare reform: California religious community capacity study.* San Francisco: Institute for Nonprofit Organization Management, University of San Francisco.

Smith, S. R., & Sosin, M. R. (2001). The varieties of faith-based agencies. *Public Administration Review, 61,* 651-670.

Unruh, H. R., & Sider, R. J. (2005). *Saving souls, serving society: Understanding the faith factor in church-based social ministry.* New York: Oxford University Press.

Vidal, A. C. (2001). *Faith-based organizations in community development.* Washington DC: The Urban Institute. Retrieved December 12, 2005, from www.huduser.org/publications/pdf/faithbased.pdf

Wiener, S. J., Kirsch, A. D., & McCormack, M. T. (2002). *Balancing the scales: Measuring the roles and contributions of nonprofit organizations and religious congregations.* Washington DC: Independent Sector.

Wind, J., & Lewis, J. W. (1994). *American congregations.* Vol. 2, *New Perspectives in the Study of Congregations.* Chicago: University of Chicago Press.

Woolever, C., & Bruce, D. (2002). *A field guide to U. S. congregations: Who's going where and why.* Louisville: Westminster John Knox.

Working Group on Human Needs and Faith-Based and Community Initiatives. (2002). *Finding common ground: 29 recommendations of the working group on human needs and faith-based and community initiatives.* Washington DC: Search for Common Ground.

Wuthnow, R. (1990). Religion and the voluntary spirit in the United States: Mapping the terrain. In R. Wuthnow & V. Hodgkinson (Eds.), *Faith and philanthropy in America.* San Francisco, CA: Jossey-Bass.

Wuthnow, R. (2004). *Saving America? Faith-based services and the future of civil society.* Princeton, NJ: Princeton University Press.

Chapter 3

Detecting and Decomposing the "Faith Factor" in Social-Service Provision and Absorption

George M. von Furstenberg

SUMMARY. Faith-based provision and reception of social services may yield results that differ either randomly or persistently (via "fixed effects") from the outcomes achieved under non-faith-based, but certainly not value-free, administration of these services. Yet attributing raw differences in performance to unobservable factors assumed to derive from "faith" should be a last resort. Instead, the objective of analysis should be to identify any such factors and their cost and strength operationally so that they can become a managed part of any program offered by existing providers or entrants.

These factors, or the cost effectiveness of employing them, could differ between secular and faith-based providers. Then members of the two groups optimally would use a different mix of means even if they were to pursue precisely the same ends. Yet program design and operation by both groups would stand to benefit from knowing the keys to their relative performance in particular areas of social service with particular groups of clients. Comparing the outcomes of experiments based on

---

George M. von Furstenberg, PhD, is J.H. Rudy Professor of Economics, Indiana University, Bloomington, IN 47405 (E-mail: vonfurst@indiana.edu).

He is indebted to the editors of this volume for many improvements.

[Haworth co-indexing entry note]: "Detecting and Decomposing the 'Faith Factor' in Social-Service Provision and Absorption." von Furstenberg, George M. Co-published simultaneously in *Journal of Religion & Spirituality in Social Work* (The Haworth Pastoral Press, an imprint of The Haworth Press, Inc.) Vol. 25, No. 3/4, 2006, pp. 39-61; and: *Faith-Based Social Services: Measures, Assessments, and Effectiveness* (ed: Stephanie C. Boddie, and Ram A. Cnaan) The Haworth Pastoral Press, an imprint of The Haworth Press, Inc., 2006, pp. 39-61

random assignment may provide little help in that regard. Micro-simulations may provide a superior approach to tightening the link between input-based model predictions and continuous learning from outcomes.

KEYWORDS. Program evaluation, social services, faith-based organizations, faith factor, fixed effects, experimental methods, microsimulations

Thus the unicorn earned a permanent place in the Bible, which later served as irrefutable proof of its existence, and an important role in most subsequent Christian writing, where the unicorn was firmly identified with Christ.–A. Salvatore (1998, p. 21)

And he said to the woman, Thy faith hath saved thee: go in peace.–Luke 7:50 (the context is inner transformation and forgiveness of sins or spiritual healing)

And he said unto her, Daughter, be of good comfort: thy faith hath made thee whole; go in peace.–Luke 8:48 (transformation through faith and healing of an untreatable blood disorder)

And Jesus said unto him, Receive thy sight: Thy faith hath saved thee.–Luke 19:42 (all: King James version)

These two sets of quotes show that assertions about the effectiveness of faith can range from (1) claims requiring the suspension of disbelief and denying the need for proof even in mundane matters that are entirely open to factual determination to (2) identifying intrinsic motivation to transform one's life as a gift of faith to oneself as if bootstrapping by the grace of God.[1] Any dispassionate examination of the operation of the faith factor in the provision and absorption of social services that respects accepted rules of evidence has to stay well away from the first type of claims that are false within their chosen terms of reference, without however precluding discernment of the power of intrinsic motivation that does not depend on physical reality. It is obviously as useless to argue that the faith factor should be taken on faith as it is to argue that the unicorn must exist without a doubt because it got into (Greek and then Latin mistranslations of) the Hebrew Bible or Old Testament. By the same token, any conception, religious or otherwise, that a provider or client makes of itself, its purpose, hopes, and goals in life, and its obligations to self and others can be part of that active ingredient of human motivation that has a bearing on treatment success.

In the language and reference of England and Scotland in the 18th Century, that is less categorical than contemporary idioms, Christian religion thus may be defined as a moral science (cf. Boulding, 1970, pp. 117- 138), but it is not a political, economic, or generically social science because individual conduct, and living faith in what is not of this world are its main subjects. Section 2 considers the mission conflicts that may arise in entrusting society's business to a mix of religious and secular service organizations, as has been done for centuries (see Stradner, 1897). Distributional tensions between groups of providers are unavoidable when professional, societal, and religious visions, competencies, and goals fail to overlap completely. Section 3 elaborates on this point by noting that mission conflicts and disagreement on priorities extend to all who hold a stake in the supply of social services, whether directly as providers or indirectly as donors and taxpayers. In the face of these multiple constituencies, comparative evaluation of providers and programs is possible only if there is prior agreement on the standards that are to be applied to common, even if initially not fully shared, objectives. Assuming these enabling conditions for evaluation are satisfied, the remainder of the paper then considers how the faith factor can be substantiated on which claims of comparative advantage of faith-based over other providers of social services often rest.

Here it appears that if the faith factor is to be operationally useful for program design and operation, it must first be taken out of the box of purely divine or religious attributions of effectiveness, such as faith and grace, and be held up to the search light in which demonstrable links and channels of transmission can become visible. In other words, the faith factor, once detected, must be decomposed into its active and humanly manageable ingredients for the programs at hand. Indeed, identifying a residual difference due to unknown causes as revealing the operation of the faith factor is just an arbitrary label for forces unknown until consequences of faith for effectiveness and efficiency can be deduced and substantiated in operational detail.

To determine how usable attributes of the faith factor may be established and employed in the design, funding, and administration of social-service programs thus involves at least two distinct steps. The first involves establishing that there is differential treatment success that could arguably be attributed to a faith factor. Section 4 shows that many existing studies erroneously stop at this point, content either to have found some such residual difference or a lack thereof. In fact, however, if the pre-qualification test regarding the *possible* existence of such factor has been met, the real work begins. As Section 5 explains, the critical next step is to model, test, and validate in detail how the faith factor arises and works. For as long as the key to this factor's effectiveness remains a mystery that keeps it out of human hands, faith must remain a speculative label for some fluid combination of effects whose past and future source, and hence future force, is unknown. Section 6 concludes.

CAN RELIGION PROVIDE TOOLS FOR SELF-IMPROVEMENT AND SOCIAL CHANGE?

Should a concrete picture emerge of how faith works to enhance the effectiveness of social services, there would still be questions about the general applicability and replicability of what has been learned. For instance, setting aside issues of publicly-funded establishment of religion, the question may arise whether religious faith can be instrumentalized without losing its power of transformation. Promoting faith on utilitarian or behaviorist grounds "because it is good for you and for society" may jeopardize the effectiveness of the faith factor for lack of intrinsic religious motivation. Intrinsic motivation leads to committing to an activity or belief system out of spontaneous choice or dedication and inner conviction not motivated by thought of recompense or of punishment and peer-group pressure avoided. Being healed on account of one's faith is orders apart from adopting a religious belief *in order* to be healed. If the "cash value" sought of religion consists of what it does for individual and social welfare (see Brennan & Waterman, 1994, p. 9), religion motivated in this extrinsic way may be debased.

Major religions and mainline congregations define social obligations and proper attitudes toward one's neighbor and require or encourage acts of charity. But they do not promulgate a clear and effective social program or offer an inclusive vision of the just society or of policies needed to achieve poverty-reduction on this earth. In this sense they lack social-policy agency for society at large. Thus, as a Catholic I may note that even those papal encyclicals, such as *Rerum Novarum* (1891), that deal explicitly with issues of social justice rarely stray far from reflecting the communalist yearning of their time without a concrete transformational, let alone effectively revolutionary, intent. The famous American economist, Frank Knight, even held that the Christian love-ethic was at best irrelevant, and at worst positively evil, with regard to the choice of social institutions essential to insuring that individual actions contribute to the general good (Emmett, 1994, pp. 109-111).

Max Weber, on the other hand, deduced an achievement-ethic based on individual empowerment and self-improvement from the Protestant Reformation that gave religious convictions a much more foundational role in the economic order of (capitalist) society. There is no question that religious beliefs, to the extent they permeate business ethics, interpersonal relations, and sense of self, can affect production and consumption of social services. Guiso, Sapienza and Zingales (2003) have re-examined the evidence linking religion, economic attitudes, income distribution, and economic growth more broadly. The subsequent discussion will be restricted to operational and evidentiary detail of the faith factor in social service programs. Although one may chafe at the inadequacy of such a restricted subject matter for the design of social policy and for evaluations of effectiveness in addressing social problems as a whole, this is the constraint under which we will proceed. Hence there will be no consideration of the links between social policies, the number of persons needing or seeking help, and the reaction of social-service providers to increased case loads that is evident for example from the following finding, "FBOs are significantly more likely to have tightened eligibility criteria since Indiana's welfare reform was adopted in 1995" (Pirog & Reingold, 2002, p. 23).

Short of a survey of religious attitudes such as that recently provided by Green (2004) with some quite uncharitable (pp. 19-30) results, there is no sure telling how religious orientation, work ethic, and bigotry mix in any country at a particular time, or whether doing more, or less, for "minorities" or "the disadvantaged" is perceived to be the way of God.

EVALUATION DEFICIT AND ITS CAUSES

"Many reasons are given for the current effort to make faith-based providers a larger part of the government-funded social safety net. The most prominent is a belief that religious providers are more effective than their secular counterparts. This is a belief that has never been tested–indeed, there is comparatively little research on the efficacy of social welfare programs in general" (Deb & Jones, 2003, p. 57). The

GAO (2002, p. 17) provides the same laconic assessment. Presumptive comparators, many "religiously non-expressive" (see Green & Sherman, 2002, p. 23) providers of social services which have been funded for decades, "continue to receive federal funding and have never been evaluated" either (Johnson, 2002, p. 22).

Unless prodded by notoriety about some program, there appears to be little political inclination or capacity of units of government to evaluate the programs they support. Saperstein (2000) worried that public accountability mandates, while being necessary for those who receive government funding, can be implemented only at the expense of the cherished autonomy of religious entities in the choice of methods applied and outcomes sought. This led him to caution religiously expressive organizations against accepting government funds for social services too readily. Others might see social benefit in their doing so because it would increase the contracting pool and the range of useful experimentation with secular and faith-based approaches and facilitate cross-fertilization between the different programs on a shared playing field. Yet Glenn (2000, p. 192) argued that the detached style that goes with professional norms "is very different from that practiced–with positive results–in many religious and quasi-religious organizations" and thus to be avoided. Still others (e.g., Light, 2000) have recommended a shift of emphasis away from final-stage compliance and performance accountability, with its focus on provider competition and client outcomes, toward a capacity-building model of accountability that focuses more on essential preparatory steps, resource inventories and qualifications. In all these instances, program evaluation, particularly by the government or third parties, and faith-based organizations do not mix easily. Hence imposition of outcome-evaluation and follow-up mandates on such organizations is likely to be politically resisted. In fact, few social-service organizations, faith-based or secular, welcome credible outcome evaluations for their own reasons, although Fischer (2005) argued that they should.

In the area of social service, program results tend to be complex and difficult to measure objectively and/or to analyze and interpret (see Blasi, 2002, p. 535). Yet even if one could obtain all the desired measures, different outcome components would be valued very differently and for different reasons by clients, assorted providers and sponsors. Although the agents that deliver social services may be nonprofits or for-profits, the fact that most social services, just like primary and secondary education in many cases, are not sold to their recipients, but granted to them, fundamentally affects every aspect of their provision. Recipients may have little influence on the volume and variety of social services provided for them via the political and administrative processes to which they are subjected. Providers, including various levels of government, have their own agendas and constraints, and financial resources may be obtained from not only government contracts but also private sources solicited by social-service providers themselves.

What Society and Clients Want from Social Services: The Best for You or Me?

Section 104 of P.L. 104-193, the Welfare Reform Act of 1996 that now bears the politically attractive label, "Charitable Choice," has more to do with providers' choices for clients than with clients' own choices. The dominant purpose of this and subsequent legislation is to allow states to contract with religious organizations on the same basis as with any other nongovernmental providers "without impairing the religious character of such organizations, and without diminishing the religious freedom of beneficiaries assisted under such programs" (Sec. 104.1.a). Other than affording an inevitably capacity-constrained choice between religious and other providers of social services, there is nothing in the legislation that refers to client satisfaction as an element relevant for the design of social services and the nature of the treatments provided.

Although it is obviously difficult to treat reluctant or dissatisfied clients successfully, the extent to which client satisfaction should rule is a matter of debate in areas where a transformation of preferences through social intervention is intended. At one end, client satisfaction with social services is irrelevant for social policy to the extent it derives from principally private benefits to the individual, such as greater social pretense and prestige outlined by Boddie & Smith (2005), the acquisition of which much of society would decline to subsidize. Client satisfaction is equally subordinate at the other end if clients are deemed incompetent, on account of youth, extreme old age, addiction, mental illness, or "moral depravity," either to judge or properly to appreciate any benefits, public or private. In between there is a vast area with considerable overlap between privately- and socially-perceived benefits. In that area, private preferences that are revealed through self-selection even in non-voucher-type programs can provide important clues to social benefits. While often complicating comparative evaluation, self-selection is likely to increase client satisfaction and hence treatment success without requiring the expenditure of additional resources. Government-endowed funds, grants from which are awarded at wide discretion, such as the Compassion Capital Fund in the U.S. Department of Health and Human Services or the Futurebuilders investment fund in the United Kingdom (see HM Treasury, 2003), help distance the funding mechanism from an immediately accountable social purpose and from government control of outcomes by citing the need for novel approaches and experimentation.

Disagreements over what should be valued and by how much thus can lead to large variations in the benefits looked for in a particular program. Both altruistic and self-interested utilitarian motives generally play some part in making the case for government-supported as well as privately-supported programs. However, it is likely that the altruistic motivation is more prominent in privately-supported programs, particularly faith-based program direction that aims to deliver good deeds to those being served. Beneficial consequences for the rest of society may be quite secondary in the charitable motivation. Some faith-based providers may also not subscribe to the efficiency principle of selecting clients on the basis of achieving the greatest discounted present value of expected benefits per unit of cost. Rather, the moral imperatives of their charitable missions, as in the ministry of Mother Teresa, may direct them to the very neediest, least tractable, or even terminal cases, and not to shoring up their remaining "useful economic life." Hence, the missions recognized by government agencies, secular non-profits, and faith-based providers of social services may differ in their emphasis on the individual being aided and why she or he is being assisted. Providers in each set will tend to evaluate outcomes according to their particular sense of mission and of human worth or dignity.

Because they pursue objectives that are at least in part different from those of others, faith-based providers may also employ a somewhat different mix of means to achieve them. Since their focus is more on saving the individual in trouble than saving society from that person, a firm faith commitment may appear as a powerful tool for achieving a permanent change in behavior primarily for the spiritual, social, and economic good of that individual. By the same token, those disinclined to make such a faith commitment would require different treatment approaches for maximum benefit if the faith factor works only for the faithful and cannot be made to work for those of little faith. Alternatively, faith-based providers of social services may claim that the faith factor operates primarily through them and their religiously-based communication, care, and motivation skills, i.e., mostly from the supply rather than the demand side. In that case faith-based organizations could turn in a superior record even if they treated the same cross-section of clients as other organizations and no self-selection by religious preference or match-up between clients and providers were allowed.

Prerequisites for Accountability

Given this welter of special circumstances and special pleading, comparative evaluation is possible only if there is agreement on common standards to be applied to objectives that are weighted and scored under a scheme with often multiple objectives adopted in advance. If program operators were free to apply their own diagnostic, rules of evidence, and choice and weighting of objectives for scoring the outcomes of their services unchallenged, evaluation would be thwarted for lack of a common reference. Substituting a multiplicity of private and parochial visions for a shared public vision of the appropriate policy objectives and service benefits, just like differences in public/private visions, would complicate appropriate program design and evaluation. To reduce this lack of accountability, government contracts often seek to mandate the performance of specific functions that are entirely funded with public means. In the final analysis, there must be prior agreement on outcome criteria and measures if professional evaluations are to help determine what it is in faith-based and other forms of administration that contributes to greater or lesser success in particular areas. The pursuit of outcomes so vague and variable that they can not be evaluated should not be eligible for public funding.

Evaluation with consequences for the allocation of public and private funds thus not only helps maintain, but creates quality by defending competitive selection under common standards against privileged selection under "unique" standards, i.e., no standards at all. To achieve comparability on any set of multiple outcome and input scales does involve some sacrifice of context and of a ready means of taking account of special factors or genuine elements of experimentation and uniqueness, but a modest loss of fit may be less damaging than the consequences of failure to evaluate at all. Hence I turn to the two stages of evaluation which the faith factor must pass before it can contribute to the quality of supply and absorption of social services in a demonstrable, and hence operationally useful, way.

STEP 1:
ESTABLISHING WHETHER FAITH
MAY BE THE UNOBSERVED, RESIDUAL FACTOR
IN ACCOUNTING FOR DIFFERENCES IN PERFORMANCE
OF SOCIAL SERVICE PROGRAMS AND THEIR CLIENTS

Assuming that the conditions that permit comparative evaluation have been met, the faith factor can show signs first of its existence and then of its usability only by clearing two successive hurdles. The first of these, which is treated in this section, is this: *If the faith factor is to have any substantive content, it must be possible to reject the Null hypothesis that faith and being faith-based per se have nothing to do with any differences in treatment success that may be observed between different organizations.* Provided this Null can be rejected for a particular set of programs and their providers, the next questions, left for Section 5, relate to the content of the faith factor and to what any measurable consequences of that factor are due.

In some, perhaps many, cases differences in outcomes[2] between faith-based and other providers of social services have little or nothing to do with faith per se because alternative explanations are quite sufficient to account for the differences observed. Consider, for instance, the case where faith-based providers appear to perform less well in certain regards than others. Kennedy (2003) did not jump from this result to deploring the waste of resources that appears to be associated with the use of prayers and supplications as motivational and treatment devices compared with other approaches to get at the problem. Instead she checked whether performance-depressing attributes that have a merely incidental and unsystematic correlation with faith-based providers could have handicapped the latter's performance temporarily. In the end she allowed that the difference in outcomes may have nothing to do with faith at all because there may be an "inexperienced newcomer effect" that has escaped complete statistical standardization. That effect could wear off as experience and more connections with quality employers are acquired by new faith-based providers:

In Indiana, in a comparison of the outcomes of job training and placement efforts of faith-based and secular organizations, secular organizations had somewhat better results. Persons trained and placed by secular organizations garnered more hours of work; they were also more likely to get jobs offering health insurance benefits. It is important to note, however, that the religious organizations in this study tended to be relatively new to government contracting. They were also much smaller than the secular contractors. While the analysis is controlled for these variables, it is still possible that with increased experience, the gap between the two types of organizations would narrow or disappear. (p. 93)

The CARA Program

Conversely, there are arguably faith-based programs elsewhere that have done exceptionally well by building broad-based support from civil society, political heavyweights, and business into a dense network of relationships with high-quality employers. One of these is The CARA Program (TCP), based in Chicago. It is non-denominationally religious in that each day all CARA participants share a "motivation" or prayer that is designed to reinforce their self-esteem and enhance their focus on achieving positive goals for their families.

For individuals to be eligible for the program they must be homeless and/or "at risk," drug free for at least 4 months and pass a drug test, mentally stable not further defined, able to work (i.e., with access to childcare, having an ID card), and motivated and able to demonstrate their desire to return to self-sufficiency. An individual's readiness is assessed after the initial contact meeting. Since 1991, TCP has served over 2,000 homeless and at-risk individuals, with over 1,000 of those achieving full-time employment with benefits. Of those admitted to the program, almost three-quarters were women, 27 percent had no high school diploma or GED, 36 percent had one or more previous convictions, and 60 percent came from homeless shelters or recovery facilities. The average hourly wage of program graduates then working was $9.74 in 2002 not counting wage supplements, and the 12-month job-retention rate of participants was 68 percent at their initial placement, and 78 percent overall (with or without a change in employer).[3] Permanent job placement is with "approximately 90 CARA companies." After first placement, TCP staff and volunteers continue to counsel participants on problems from goal-setting and budgeting to job-advancement and housing. Other resources provided by TCP to employed participants include financial assistance for rent and transportation, matched-saving plan, housing referrals, homeownership opportunities, free legal and dental-care assistance, and clothing.

The program's Web site, *www.thecaraprogram.org*, thus describes a program with a proud and incentive-compatible record of achievement in that some of the funding it receives is dependent on placement and retention of its clients in living-wage jobs. However, selection and retention criteria and what they imply about the comparability of reported success rates with those of other programs are not fully explained. To what extent are capacity constraints binding so that a high level of selectivity known as cream-skimming can be practiced? If clients are selected on the basis of likelihood to succeed prior to any treatment-induced transformation, are they dropped as soon as they show signs of failing to live up to that promise? These and other relevant questions, for instance about the cost of the program and the reasons for its high civic visibility and business and political support, are not answered on the Web site. The point is that neither the Chicago-based nor the Indianapolis-based programs can bring out the workings or failures of the faith factor, pure and simple. While client motivation obviously matters, faith is only one of its possible sources, and the outcomes in both locations appear to be quite explicable without needing to be attributed to faith or religious practices.

Selection Bias in Experimental Designs

It is also extremely difficult to avoid biasing outcomes through self-selection. Obviously it would be pointless to compare the outcomes of faith-based social service programs that have only co-religionists as clients with programs that serve a representative cross-section of religious and non-religious clients. If providers who share basic social, ethical, cultural, and religious convictions and ethnic identities, whatever they are, find it easier to communicate and to understand each other than providers and clients who come from different "planets," then the degree of homogeneity of providers and clients is positively associated with treatment success. Again in this case no reference to faith as such would be warranted.

To eliminate this crude form of selection bias, Fischer (2005) attempted to experiment within self-selected groups to overcome the problem of assigning subjects randomly to alternative forms of treatment, some of which they may regard as far less agreeable than others. Having first sorted individuals according to their express preference for inclusion in faith-disposed, faith-indifferent, or faith-averse treatment groups, he would randomly assign members of each group to sub-groups, locally varying the religious intensity of the preferred type of treatment without changing its basic orientation. Faith-disposed individuals, for instance, would be randomly assigned to two faith-based program alternatives that differed in their religious intensity. The goal of the randomized experiment would be to determine which of the two chosen levels of intensity works better in this group.

Under certain assumptions such an experiment could fail to provide information on the efficacy of alternative treatments within the group no matter what its outcome and provide only information on the composition of that group. Take as the null hypothesis that clients of faith-based, like of other social service programs generally know best what manner of service delivery works for them. Then those who get treated in the manner they prefer (at given shadow supply prices or resource costs per treatment) stand to reap greater treatment benefits than those subjected to an equally expensive form of treatment less favored. The upshot is that nothing might be learned from the randomized experiment about differential treatment success *per se*. Rather the experiment so far may serve only to identify the unbalanced distribution of clients with regard to the relative attractiveness of the two alternative forms of treatment picked for random assignment to members of the group.

To rectify this imbalance, assume all members of the group are first asked to identify the preferred treatment in each set of hypothetical program alternatives put before them. The composition of these sets by degree of faith-intensity can then be varied until half the members of the group prefer one form of the faith-based treatment and half the other intensity being offered. Only after this advance balancing of the treatment group has been achieved can random assignment of the group's members to the two subgroups be trusted to achieve outcome-neutral stratification by client preference. Once differential treatment effects are validly discovered and become known, they will, of course, tilt the playing field for future experiments as the new information will change the distribution of preferences for different degrees of religious intensity in treatments. The formulation of relevant choices, and ultimately the composition of supply by faith-intensity, should change accordingly.

Technically, the problem for comparative evaluation is not just that variation in opportunities for self-selection–a process that arises because those who expect to benefit from a program are most likely to enroll in it–biases methods of treatment success from the start if it contributes to unobserved differences in receptivity from one treatment group to another (see Heckman, Tobias, & Vytlacil, 2001). A further obstacle to generalization now arises from clients' receptivity to treatment being dependent on the degree of religious (or nonreligious) homogeneity with the type of provider, and providers' ability to deliver effective treatments being dependent on their being of the same faith, or lack of faith, as their clients.[4] Lack of faith cannot, of course, be equated to a lack of values in treatment. Bielefeld, Littlepage and Thelin (2003, p. 81) reported for instance that there was little difference between secular and faith-based providers in appreciating the importance of instilling and strengthening values to promote their clients' success.

Nevertheless, politically, if belief systems that are shared by providers and their clients could be shown to raise responsiveness to a given treatment systematically, social service provision could become a religiously fragmented enterprise. In it clients having any particular religious conviction could be seen as entitled to providers with matching faith characteristics. In addition, "having religion" could be offered as a service qualification by providers and "getting religion" as a desideratum for clients "so that the individual could then experience a variety of benefits demonstrated in the literature on organic religion" (Fischer, 2005, MS p. 17). If represented as a professional qualification by pervasively sectarian entities, religion thus could become profoundly divisive in the conduct of social services.

What Can Be Learned from Experiments with Clients?

Biotech scientists evaluating the effect of an as yet unapproved drug can be reasonably sure that statistically significant differences, say in survival rates, can be attributed to that drug provided patients were assigned randomly to (1) a control group and (2) a treatment group, and (3) participants in this double-blind experiment were unable to infer on their own or through hints given by providers to which group they belonged.[5] Being based on response "constants" of the human organism, findings of differential effectiveness that can be replicated under identically controlled conditions with the same expected outcome but have no other substantiation thus can be used for management decisions in this area.

Experimental techniques are far less applicable and their results far less useful for management in the area of social service. In particular, there are no such things as double-blind, or even one-eyed, social-service experiments since providers know what type of service they are dispensing and clients are quite aware of what services they are actually getting though not necessarily of what else they could be getting. Not only may treatment work better for persons with one set of known characteristics than another, but subjects may self-select for a particular treatment partly because they believe in it or have private reasons and motivation that lead them to expect it to work best for them. Unlike in clinical trials, a purely empirical approach to determining what has worked best is not enough to predict future success: Future performance need not equal past performance, least of all when new entrants are involved and many constituents of success keep changing because they are poorly understood and hence not controlled. Social organizations do not mechanically produce services and their clients do not respond passively and predictably like natural organisms to the treatment offered so that its efficacy can be discovered merely by repeated application. Rather, these organizations are intentional and fluid contrivances that are designed to gear incentives, motivations, and mechanisms to achieving certain sets of objectives for certain clients under budgetary constraints. If some part of the observed differences in their degrees of success cannot be explained in any way, it helps very little to attribute these unexplained differences to "divine grace," "secular savvy," or any other self-congratulatory organizational rationale or distinction.

There is a more general lesson here. Tentative identification of the unexplained residual basically "on faith" remains of little value for funding, operation, and management decisions unless the mechanisms and any systematic correlates of faith-based provision or client reception of social services can be clarified convincingly. Because the assets and liabilities of various providers, including the composition of their staff, means of supply, and the responsiveness of their clients are far from fixed over case or time, applying labels of this kind to observed differences in performance provides no reliable guide to what to expect in the future and hence can have no operational significance. If we do not know what it is that makes a program or provider more effective, there is no way to make sure that this unknown factor is still there next year or the year after or when new programs are started and new providers enter. Rather, decoding is needed that shows how any plausibly alleged faith factor works.

STEP 2:
DETERMINING FAITH FACTOR'S MEASURABLE
ATTRIBUTES AND CONTROLLABLE CORRELATES

Assume now that the preliminary analysis in step 1 in a particular case points to differences in performance that could arguably be attributed to a "faith factor." The question then becomes exactly how this factor works and through and for whom it can be activated. Previous literature often stopped short of this critical next question. Instead it contented itself with determining whether faith-based providers are better than others in a crude group-comparison process. That process is analogous to introducing and estimating fixed effects in the econometric analysis of data panels.

In panel estimation, the size and statistical significance of fixed effects rarely is of much interest in its own right. In most econometric applications their coefficients thus are not even reported. Rather, if panels differ in characteristics that may have some influence on outcomes whose determinants are to be established, fixed effects typically are used to take out sources of heterogeneity among these panels that could bias and invalidate evidence obtained from their combination. Fixed effects thus tend to be used to achieve data comparability along other dimensions of interest and not because they are revealing of themselves. To establish the importance of the faith-factor on the other hand, the focus is on the size and significance of this fixed effect itself.

Exact identification of the pathways of effectiveness is also necessary in the evaluation of providers of social services because it helps minimizes non-operational, and therefore sterile, references to faith as an explanatory factor. Religious experiences and new-found, or rediscovered religion certainly may stimulate beneficial auto-suggestion, unleash the power of positive thinking, and instill intrinsic motivation to do things out of love of God and neighbor or because they are right, decent. Faith-based righteousness can also poison social relations and detract from the common good, but either way faith matters. Religion may be a stronger and simpler motivator when it is united with an anthropomorphic Divine Being that can take orders like "God Bless America" or prayers like "Help me find Spot," than when it is–free from any definite notion of God or theology–a measure of the limits of human knowledge. Paraphrasing Einstein's definition of his religion (see Torrance, 1997, p. 5), acknowledgment of such limits can lead to abstract veneration for anything that is beyond what we can comprehend.

Fixed and Random Effects by Provider Groups

Fixed effects in econometrics deserve no similar reverence for revealing little about their origin. Rather, large fixed effects often pose the challenge of whittling them down through decoding. If differences in outcomes between provider groups can be attributed to measurable differences in characteristics of service and in who is being served, there may be no otherwise inexplicable residual to be attributed to the grouping criterion–faith-based or other provider–per se. An otherwise unexplained group-systematic residual would be revealed by the mean of the residuals estimated differing significantly from zero for one or more groups. However, rather than focusing on differences in these means of residuals between groups per se, the econometric purpose of adjusting for them usually lies elsewhere as shown by the following quote:

> In Classical econometrics, 'fixed' effects are treated as parameters and estimated by a least-squares dummy variable . . . 'Random' effects are assimilated to the error term and estimated by generalized least squares . . . In both instances, effects are basically treated as errors: "the use of dummy variables is an attempt to specify a model with an error term that indeed has zero mean" . . . That is, effects are 'nuisance' or 'incidental' parameters, which may distort a consistent estimate of the slope. (Rendón, 2002, p. 2)

In a random effects model the residual performance components that are common to each group but distinct between them change randomly over time. Then cross-sectional comparisons of performance between faith-based and other groups that implicitly assume fixed, i.e., constant rather than just randomly fluctuating, group-specific effects could generate a bewildering variety of results, with successive analyses producing inconsistent findings. Of course, neither fixed nor random effects analysis by itself can show how the faith factor functions, in which environment it works best, and whether it can be activated and used in design, management, and day-to-day operation of social-service programs. Rather, choosing the correct stochastic representation for group-specific (symmetric) residual effects and for the individual (idiosyncratic) program or client "noise" that surrounds them at a point in time is important for efficient and unbiased estimation of the effect of decision and control variables associated with program management.

Simulation Approaches to Determining Operation and Content of the Faith Factor

The econometric approach to determining the contribution of a particular intervention or group difference while also guarding against evaluation bias in assessing this contribution is to include all those factors which a model or conjecture identifies as possibly contributing to differences in outcomes between those with or without the particular intervention or faith-based manner of treatment. The efficiency of econometric estimates and hence their statistical significance tends to suffer when there are high degrees of correlation between explanatory variables or between them and the grouping criterion. However, the entire thrust of econometric analysis is to let observed correlations between the grouping criterion and explanatory variables help explain why crude differences in group performance may be very different from the adjusted differences revealed by econometric analysis. The analytical objective is to understand why there are differences in performance between providers distinguished by the grouping criterion. It is not just to establish that there *are* such differences when all other explanatory factors that are deemed relevant to performance have been randomized, as in the experimental analyses discussed before.

Micro-simulations can provide additional insights for policy planning by modeling the effectiveness of alternative program designs in view of suitably constrained optimization behavior by providers and clients. Such simulations can be useful first for *ex ante* or provisional evaluations which experimental approaches cast as pilot programs may provide as well. Secondly, micro-simulations can provide a firm grasp on the outcomes to be expected from any adopted design. These expectations can then be contrasted with subsequent results for either model-policy validation or revision in a process of continuous learning.

The evaluation techniques developed for micro-simulations have been applied broadly to social programs only since the 1990s, nationally in part under the auspices of the National Research Council (e.g., Citro & Hanushek, 1991) and internationally by the World Bank.[6] Researchers using micro-simulations attempt to determine the complex effects of programs *ex ante* through the construction and simulation of behavioral models. They do so most commonly by using some form of CGE (computable general equilibrium) technique. Relevant econometric evidence or response variables obtained from earlier studies are used to calibrate such models. Like actual pilot programs, micro-simulations are used to provide real-time help with design and choice of any new programs before costly commitments are made that are difficult to reverse or to redirect in midcourse. Because they provide truly out-of-sample predictions of effects, the outcomes of the micro-simulation exercises can be confirmed or challenged by the evidence that subsequently accrues from programs that are adopted. Macro-simulations may provide the overarching systemic framework in which the investigation of the micro effects of a program is embedded, particularly if that program is part of a broader social-policy package.

CONCLUSION

The evaluation of social programs and all their competing providers is necessary for quality control and for improvement through continuous review of each program's intermediate targets and ultimate goals and the best ways to achieve them. So far, however, comparative studies of possible differences in the effectiveness of faith-based and other providers of social services have rarely attempted to go beyond the primitive stage of finding statistically significant differences in effectiveness between the two modes or modalities of provision for reasons unknown. Only by understanding the factors contributing to these differences from the side of both providers and clients can one learn "what to do" with any such finding in terms of contract specifics, management techniques, provider and client selection, and grant support.

Both politics and performance often have an important influence on the division of roles between secular and faith-based providers of social services. As in the back and forth of European history since the late Middle Ages,[7] the boundaries between faith-based and secular care providers have shifted markedly in the United States from time to time. The tilt toward faith-based providers toward the end of the 20th and into the 21st century occurred not on the basis of superior performance already demonstrated by the advancing side but through changes in the dominant ideology and gains in the political power of churches and those eager to represent the claims of faith-based groups. It remains to be seen whether the shift toward qualifying many more faith-based providers will result in superior performance leaving aside the question of whether the lives of the needy populations as a whole, and not just of program participants, are in fact going to be improved.

To yield practical insights that can be acted upon, research must proceed to determine whether there are replicable, and hence manageable and controllable, factors that contribute to differences in performance between groups, and what these factors are. Indeed, even if there are no statistically significant differences in net outcomes in relation to inputs between faith-based and other providers at all, the reason may not be that the two types of providers really are interchangeable and do the same thing with the same types of clients. If they do in fact employ different approaches and means, then some of their service "modules" may do better and others worse to produce the overall stand-off. Hence the programs of both types of providers could be improved if they would be able to share what has been found to work best for each of them.

Just as lack of evaluation with budgetary consequences encourages fraud and waste, false evaluations can misdirect resources, hurting the intended beneficiaries of social programs. Careful modeling of the underlying sources of bias and randomness serves to reveal the strong assumptions and specification choices made, and omissions and compromises tolerated, when trying to combine unbiasedness with tractability in particular cases. It thereby implicitly cautions against overly broad or categorical generalizations. At the same time, the resulting transparency of evaluation raises the potential contribution of evaluation analysis to cumulative learning about the appropriate management and design of social service in specific settings for particular groups of clients. Confronting detailed sets of "priors" obtained from micro-simulations with evidence subsequently derived from actual program operation may be especially valuable in that regard.

NOTES

1. *Intrinsic* motivation here could arise out of love for God. It would then be based on faith in God and not on hoping for miracle cures or other self-serving ends to be advanced by the instrument of faith. By contrast, *extrinsic* motivation is derived from punishments and rewards "incentivizing" choices not made for their own sake. For contributions to the theory of self-determination in a variety of social- and personal-choice settings see Deci and Ryan (2004).

2. Hatry (1999, pp. 21-22) has defined *outcomes* as not what the program itself did (i.e., its outputs) but the consequences of what the program did. While certain program outputs, such as providing food and shelter for a person on a given day, may be necessary for achieving outcomes such as that person's becoming employed and then remaining self-supporting, outputs are not sufficient for achieving the outcomes that are the measure of performance.

3. Deb and Jones (2003, p. 61) report much lower results for another welfare-to-work program: "In the full sample (with FaithWorks), 36 percent of clients who engaged in job training were placed in jobs subsequent to training. Those who were

placed earned an average of $6.87 per hour and worked an average of 31.4 hours per week. Fifteen percent of these individuals were offered health insurance plans."

4. Matched estimator techniques also could not be applied using similarity of pre-established unconditional receptivity indexes or "propensity scores" if these scores (see Rosenbaum and Rubin, 1983) are themselves conditional on the type of organization that offers the treatment, with some favoring and others disliking a particular type. Brooks (2004) uses an econometric approach to estimate a propensity for making donations in neighborhoods with different socio-economic characteristics which then serves as the benchmark for scoring fundraising success. He notes that this propensity may not be unconditional so that fundraising prowess established by an organization in one demographic, economic, and religious environment may not be transferable to another.

5. In proposing a natural experiment to determine differences in the effectiveness of alternative treatments for substance abuse, Cnaan (2005) has tried to emulate this clinical design. However, the fact that clients are aware of the treatment they are getting and may like to have a choice in the matter complicates the interpretation of results. If providing choice and allowing self-selection are efficient along "market" lines, adding religious-intensive treatment to the mix of programs offered where it has been lacking would be beneficial, just as it would have been beneficial to add secular treatment to the mix of options where it had been denied (as in much of continental Europe up to three centuries ago). The faith factor per se is not involved.

6. A record of sometimes well-documented studies has accumulated rapidly in areas such as childhood education and job training under the auspices of the LACEA/WB/IDB Network on Inequality and Poverty. Members of this network have been working with countries, academic researchers, aid agencies and NGOs to build and test various techniques and tools that evaluate the poverty and distributional impact of economic policy choices. See the "Toolkit" http://www.worldbank.org/poverty/psia/tools.htm and Bourguignon and Pereira da Silva (2003).

7. At the time, guilds and municipalities began to establish new facilities specializing on medical services that competed successfully with religiously-based "hospitals" that had combined the practice of medicine with catering to a host of other welfare and relief functions. See Stradner (1897, pp. 135-136).

REFERENCES

Bielfeld, W., Littlepage, L., & Thelin, R. (2003). Organizational analysis: The influence of faith on impact service providers. In S. S. Kennedy & W. Bielefeld, *Charitable choice: First results from three states* (pp. 65-86). Center for Urban Policy and the Environment, School of Public and Environmental Affairs, Indiana University–Purdue University, Indianapolis.

Blasi, G. J. (2002). Government contracting and performance measurement in human services. *International Journal of Public Administration, 25* (4), 519-538.

Boddie, S. C., & Smith, R. D. (2005). Where to turn: How do public housing residents view congregation-based services?

Boulding, K. E. (1970). *Economics as a science.* New York: McGraw-Hill.

Bourguignon, F., & Pereira da Silva, L. A. (Eds.). (2003). *The impact of economic policies on poverty and income distribution: Evaluation techniques and tools.* Washington and New York: A co-publication of the World Bank and Oxford University Press.

Brennan, H. G., & Waterman, A. M. C. (Eds.). (1994). *Economics and religion: Are they distinct?* Boston: Kluwer Academic.

Brooks, A. C. (2004). Evaluating the effectiveness of nonprofit fundraising. *Policy Studies Journal 32*, 363-374.

Citro, C .F., & Hanushek, E. A. (Eds.). (1991). *Improving information for social policy decisions: The uses of microsimulation modeling.* Vol. I: *Review and recommendations*, Vol. II: *Technical papers.* Washington, DC: National Academy Press. (Panel to Evaluate Microsimulation Models for Social Welfare Programs, Committee on National Statistics, Commission on Behavioral and Social Sciences and Education, National Research Council.)

Cnaan, R. A. (2005). Social service research and religion: Thoughts about how to measure intervention-based impact. *This volume.*

Deb, P., & Jones, D. (2003). Does faith work? A preliminary comparison of labor market outcomes of job training programs. In S. S. Kennedy & W. Bielefeld, *Charitable choice: First results from three states* (pp. 57-64). Center for Urban Policy and the Environment, School of Public and Environmental Affairs, Indiana University–Purdue University, Indianapolis.

Deci, E. L., & Ryan, R. M. (Eds.). (2004). *Handbook of self-determination research.* Rochester: University of Rochester Press.

Emmett, R. B. (1994). Frank Knight: Economics versus religion. In H. G. Brennan & A. M. C. Waterman, (Eds.), *Economics and religion: Are they distinct?* (103-120). Boston: Kluwer Academic.

Fischer, R. L. (2005). Confounded by faith: Evaluation research in faith-based organizations. *Evaluation & Program Planning*, forthcoming.

GAO (U.S. General Accounting Office). (2002). *Charitable choice: Overview of research findings on implementation.* GAO-02-337, Washington, DC.

Glenn, C. L. (2000). *The ambiguous embrace: Government and faith-based schools and social agencies.* Princeton, NJ: Princeton University Press.

Green, J. C. (2004). *The American religious landscape and political attitudes: A baseline for 2004.* The Pew Forum on Religion and Public Life. www.pewforum.org/publications/surveys/green-full.pdf

Green, J. C., & Sherman, A. (2002). *Fruitful collaborations: A survey of government-funded faith-based programs in 15 states.* Charlottesville VA: Hudson Institute.

Guiso, L., Sapienza, P., & Zingales, L. (2003). People's opium? Religion and economic attitudes, *Journal of Monetary Economics, 50* (1), 225-282.

Hatry, H. P. (1999). *Performance management: Getting results.* Washington, DC: The Urban Institute.

Heckman, J., Tobias, J. L., & Vytlacil, E. (2001). *Four parameters of interest in the evaluation of social programs.* Draft, University of Chicago, June 19.

HM Treasury, Compact Working Group. (2003). *Futurebuilders: An investment fund for voluntary and community sector public service delivery.* Norwich: Controller of

Her Majesty's Stationary Office, September. Accessible through www.hm-treasury. gov.uk

Johnson, B. R. (2002). *Objective hope, assessing the effectiveness of faith-based organizations: A review of the literature.* Philadelphia: Center for Research on Religion and Urban Civil Society (CRRUCS Report), University of Pennsylvania.

Kennedy, S. S. (2003). Preliminary Conclusions. In S.S. Kennedy & W. Bielfeld, 93-97.

Kennedy, S. S., & Bielefeld, W. (2003). *Charitable choice: First results from three states.* Center for Urban Policy and the Environment, School of Public and Environmental Affairs, Indiana University–Purdue University, Indianapolis.

Light, P. C. (2000). *Making nonprofits work: A report on the tides of nonprofit management reform.* Washington, DC: The Brookings Institution.

Pirog, M., & Reingold, D. A. (2002). Has the social safety net been ALTAred? New roles for faith-based organizations. *Perspectives.* Occasional Series, Bloomington: Office of the Dean, School of Public and Environmental Affairs, Indiana University.

Razin, A., Rubinstein, Y., & Sadka, K. (2004). Fixed costs and FDI: The conflicting effects of productivity shocks. National Bureau of Economic Research Working Paper 10864.

Rendón, S. (2002). Fixed and Random Effects in Classical and Bayesian regression. Working Paper 02-15, Economics Series 03, Department of Economics, Universidad Carlos III de Madrid.

Rosenbaum, P. R., & Rubin, D. B. (1983). The central role of propensity score in observational studies for causal effects. *Biometrika, 70,* 41-55.

Salvatore. A. (1998). *The unicorn tapestries at the Metropolitan Museum of Art.* New York: H. M. Abrams.

Saperstein, D. (2003). Public accountability and faith-based organizations: A problem best avoided. *Harvard Law Review, 116,* 1353-1396.

Stradner, A. (1897). *Das sociale Wirken der katholischen Kirche in Oesterreich, II. Band: Diocese Seckau (Herzogthum Steiermark).* Vienna: Commissions-Verlag von Mayer & Co. Available in Bibliotheca Admontensis, Stift Admont, Austria.

Torrance, T. (1997). Einstein and God. Center for Theological Inquiry. http://www.ctinquiry. org/publications/reflections_volume_1/torrance.htm

Chapter 4

Faith-Based Programs
and the Role of Empirical Research

Bruce A. Thyer

SUMMARY. After some decades of being subject to neglect or contempt, faith-based social care programs are receiving increased attention and resources enabling them to undertake a greater role in the national network of human services. Faith-based programs receiving public support can expect to be rightly scrutinized by the public, in terms of their ability to attain professed program goals. The tools of conventional empirically-oriented program evaluation research have tremendous potential to help demonstrate the effectiveness of faith-based programs, which will justify their receipt of ongoing support from public funds. Negative research findings can be properly scrutinized by the faith-based community of service providers to help make tough, data-based, decisions on funding priorities. Several examples are described, illustrating how various types of faith-based programs have profitably participated in program evaluation studies.

Bruce A. Thyer, PhD, is affiliated with the College of Social Work, Florida State University.

Address correspondence to: Bruce A. Thyer, PhD, College of Social Work, Florida State University, Tallahassee, FL 32306 (E-mail: bthyer@fsu.edu).

[Haworth co-indexing entry note]: "Faith-Based Programs and the Role of Empirical Research." Thyer, Bruce A. Co-published simultaneously in *Journal of Religion & Spirituality in Social Work* (The Haworth Pastoral Press, an imprint of The Haworth Press, Inc.) Vol. 25, No. 3/4, 2006, pp. 63-82; and: *Faith-Based Social Services: Measures, Assessments, and Effectiveness* (ed: Stephanie C. Boddie, and Ram A. Cnaan) The Haworth Pastoral Press, an imprint of The Haworth Press, Inc., 2006, pp. 63-82.

KEYWORDS. Empirical research, faith-based programs, evidence-based practice

A significant proportion of social care in the United States has long been provided by individuals and organizations who are faith-based. Indeed, in the very beginnings of social services in this country it would seem that a significant proportion of our social services were provided by non-governmental organizations affiliated with various religious groups. The significance of organized religion was recognized early on as an important influence in peoples' lives and as a potential agent for positive change. Below are listed a few representative quotes from some early social service texts which stressed the historical links between contemporary social services and its faith-based foundations:

> The commonest and most powerful incentive to benevolence has been everywhere and at all times that supplied by religion. (Warner, 1908, p. 4)

> The religious motive has always been one of the strong forces back of the impulse to social amelioration. (Todd, 1920, p. 68)

> The roots of almost all modern social work services are in religious organizations; hence the church can be considered the 'mother of social work.' (Johnson, 1941, p. 404)

The Roman Catholic church alone exerted an immense role at the national level in the provision of social care. As noted by Warner (1908, p. 377):

> In 1903, one-third of the benevolent institutions listed in the special census report, i.e., hospitals, day nurseries, permanent and temporary homes for adults and children, were under ecclesiastical control.

See also the landmark work of Lubov (1972, p. 5) who claimed that:

> Charity organization spokesmen. . . . were missionaries, in the most literal sense, of a new benevolent gospel. They viewed themselves as exponents of a holy cause, priests lighting a path to secular salvation.

As the nascent field of social service strove for public recognition as a legitimate and independent profession, one requiring undergraduate (if indeed not graduate) level education, some distancing occurred from its religious roots, in favor of a closer embrace of a more scientific orientation to social care. Richmond herself of course was an early advocate of a more scientific orientation to social work, as were later influential writers such as Grace Abbott (1931), Arthur Todd (1920), Alice Cheney (1926), and Frank Bruno (1936). It came to be seen that accepting a scientific orientation was intrinsic to efforts to professionalize social service. For example, Cheney provided the following simple definition of this field:

> All voluntary attempts to extend benefits which are made in response to a need, are concerned with social relationships, *and avail themselves of scientific knowledge and methods.* (Cheney, 1926, p. 24, italics added)

The influence of Comte's positivism was evident as social services attempted to become more scientific. In the early 1800s, as Comte conceptualized the development of the sciences in various fields, e.g., mathematics, physics, chemistry, astronomy, biology, and up to and including the study of human affairs, explanatory and interventive efforts were seen to historically evolve through three levels, the theological, the metaphysical, and the positive (see Comte, 1953; Mill, 1887; Pickering, 1993). Explanations akin to vitalism or animism were used by primitive human beings, as in thunder or plagues being caused by the anger of the gods or due to other magical or supernatural forces. Over time, these became superceded by metaphysical ones, as in the phlogiston theory of fire, the bodily humour theory of physical disease, or the etheric theory for the transmission of light, explanatory accounts involving not supernatural influences but of non-theological forces too occult or subtle to be measured by science. Over time, such metaphysical accounts were in turn superceded by causal theories involved solely natural forces, energies or laws which were capable of fairly robust demonstration via direct observation of their existence or validity. These were early on known as *positive* explanations, being based on observable, replicable, data, hence the term positivism. Indeed, Comte's original term for what he later called sociology was *social physics*, carrying with it the clear message that human affairs would ultimately be amenable to explanatory accounts as clear as those of, and derivable from, physics itself.

Frank Sanborn helped establish the American Social Science Association (ASSA) shortly after the American Civil War, an important organization whose ". . . dominant intellectual mode was a combination of idealism and positivism" (Chaiklin, 2005, p. 130). A direct offshoot of the ASSA was the Conference on Charities (in 1879), and its successors, in 1884 the National Conference on Charities and Correction (NCCC), in 1917 the National Conference on Social Work, and in 1957, the National Conference on Social Welfare, which dissolved in the 1980s (Haskell, 2000). A paper presented at the 1889 meeting of the NCCC was titled *Scientific Charity*, and an article appearing in the influential journal *The Charities Review* in 1894 was titled *A Scientific Basis for Charity* (see Thyer, 2004). Social services, for a time, actually became known as *scientific charity*, or *scientific philanthropy*, names eventually superceded by the more generic *social work*.

Comte's conceptualization, even if seen as overly simplistic and inaccurate in the light of the 21st century, nevertheless were widely embraced by the emerging field of supposedly scientific social work. See, for example, the views of Professor Stuart Alfred Queen, Professor of Sociology at Washington University:

> It is believed that by displacing theological concepts with scientific, i.e., "supernatural" and "natural," the prospects of understanding, prediction and control are considerably enhanced . . . Instead of praying for jobs and prosperity, we go in for business forecasting, consider ten-year programs of public works, solicit non-seasonal orders with long delivery time, and experiment with unemployment insurance. . . . Instead of laying the erratic and annoying behavior of some person to a wicked heart and urging him to repent, we make a careful study of his personal history and present conditions to see when and how the trouble started, and by what medical, surgical, hygienic, domestic, or other means it may be controlled . . . In a certain sense, our approach is no more moral than it is theological. (Queen, 1927, cited in Warner, Queen & Harper, 1930, p. 563)

Carol Germain (1970, p. 9) quoted Charles D. Kellogg of the Philadelphia Charity Organization Society, who said in 1880 "Charity is a science, the science of social therapeutics, and has laws like all other sciences." The influence of positivism was also evident in Mary Richmond's writings, as in "Thoughts and events are facts. The question whether a thing be fact or not is the question whether it can be affirmed with certainty" (Richmond, 1917, p. 53). Bertha Capen Reynolds also weighed in on the side of positivism:

> A second characteristic of scientifically-oriented social work is that it accepts the objective reality of forces outside itself with which it must cooperate . . . The scientific orientation demands something else, however, a price which sometimes we find hard to pay. We must give up the illusion that we ourselves are beyond the reach of a science of human relationships . . . Hardest of all is the necessity of applying scientific and not magical thinking to ourselves and to our evaluation of what we do . . . The promise in a scientifically-oriented social work lies in its unlimited capacity for growth. (Reynolds, 1942, pp. 24, 28, 30)

A clearer exposition could not be found of Comte's contention that supernatural thinking must be superceded by the reasoning of natural science. Positivism even pervaded the literary world of the mid-1800s, as in the following quote from Walt Whitman's *Song of Myself*:

> I accept Reality and dare not question it, Materialism first and last imbuing.
> Hurrah for positive science! long live exact demonstration!

The above quotes are representative of the tremendous influence Comte's positivism had across the entire spectrum of intellectual, political and academic thought in American, being seen as directly responsible for the rise of our nation's liberal and progressive movements (see Harp, 1995; Hawkins, 1936), as well as influencing social services in particular.

Ironically, a recent survey of conservative scholars by the journal *Human Events* found that Comte's seminal book *Introduction to Positive Philosophy* was rated among the top ten most *destructive* books ever published during the 19th and 20th centuries, ranked with other classics such as *The Communist Manifesto, Das Kapital, Mein Kampf,* and *Quotations from Chairman Mao,* all heady competition indeed! (See *http://humaneventsonline.com/article.php?id=7591*)

American social service workers also used the leverage of science to help improve their status as a profession. In the words of Arthur Todd:

> *. . . the scientific spirit is necessary to social work whether it is a real profession or only a go-between craft.* (Todd, 1920, p. 66, italics in original)

Faith-based social services seemingly became impaled on the twin prongs of positivism and professionalism, in that both orientations called for a repudiation of the theological in favor of the scientific, and in word, American professional social services became increasingly *secularized*.

Further impetus to this change occurred by the middle of the last century, in regards to the provision of social welfare services, spurred on by the profound reforms of the New Deal of the 1930s. Welfare services came to be more viewed as the responsibility of the state and federal governments (although America never became a welfare-state in the sense of the usual interpretation of the term), and faith-based social care became considerably less conspicuous:

> For the American mind, the private nature of religion remains unassailable, but the average citizen is willing now to tolerate the concept of an interlocking relationship between public and private efforts in all other fields. In welfare it is generally conceded that responsibility for meeting widespread and continuing needs is that of the community as a whole. (Hamilton, 1940, p. 263)

In other words, social services were not to be primarily provided by the church, temple, or synagogue, but by the state. This remains the mainstream view of early 21st century social work:

> Faith-based initiatives can provide some basic supports and the social welfare state can make use of these initiatives, but the driving force behind social change should remain the responsibility of the state. (Belcher, Fandetti, & Cole, 2004, p. 274)

But despite this seeming minimizing of faith-based programs, they have continued to soldier on, so much so that Garland noted that in 1991, churches gave an estimated $6.6 billion to social causes, and about 12% of surveyed members of the National Association of Social Workers practiced in sectarian settings (Garland, 1995). These are substantial contributions indeed from the faith-based community, and it would be inaccurate to label them as residual or ancillary.

Within the social services professions there reside continuing tensions and conflicts between the faith-based and secular constituencies. Professing to be a field which values inclusiveness and diversity, and respect for divergent points of view, many practitioners find the presence of individuals of faith in their midst, and of faith-based programs supplementing or in some cases supplanting, traditionally secular programs of social care, an uncomfortable experience, one which generates occasional points of tension. But there is more than discomfort. In some cases these secularized programs and faculty actively disparaged faith-based social service programs, or expressed negative attitudes towards the highly religious student who seeks social work degrees. It is not uncommon to find the religious views of some social service workers in the academy and in practice actively criticized by their secular colleagues (e.g., Belcher, Fandetti, & Cole, 2004; Sanzenbach, 1989; Hodge, 2002).

A political sea-change occurred with the election of George W. Bush as President. One of his early acts was to establish a White House Office of Faith-based and Community Initiatives, currently headed by Jim Towey, former Secretary for the Florida Department of Children and Family Services. The function of this office is to reduce

> . . . regulatory and policy barriers which have kept faith-based programs from partnering with the Federal government to help Americans in need. It has also worked to put into place regulations to ensure that faith-based organizations are able to compete on an equal footing for Federal funding within constitutional guidelines, without impairing the religious character of such organizations and without diminishing the religious freedom of beneficiaries. (see *www.whitehouse.gov/government/fbci/*)

It is repeatedly stressed by the White House Office in all its venues and publications that it is legitimate to fund social services, *but not* religious teaching, proselytizing, or evangelical work. For example,

> . . . government has no business funding religious worship or teaching. However, our government should support the good work of religious people who are changing America . . . (President George W. Bush, 29 October 2003, *www.whitehouse.gov/news/releases/ 2003/10/20031029-10.html*)

This approach seems both wise and legal, to the extent that it is actually adhered to.

An oft-cited focus of the Bush administration is to reduce the size of federal government. This has often taken the form of discontinuing the provision of social services using Federal or state-paid employees and systems of care, and opting instead to use Federal payments to underwrite having *private-sector providers* deliver the very same services. This has taken place across the country and involves many disparate systems of care such as the prison system, parole monitoring, child protective services, mental health care, job placement services, and substance abuse treatment. Related political concepts include *Devolution*– "The process of moving social programs from federal agencies to state agencies and from states to localities" (Barker, 2003, p. 118), and *New Federalism:*

> An ideology that advocates reducing national spending and taxation, deregulating national controls on businesses and institutions, and ceding more responsibilities to state governments. The term was used by the Reagan administration to describe some of its policies. (Barker, 2003, p. 294)

The convenient congruence between the pragmatics of providing state-support to faith-based organizations who in turn deliver social services, and the conservative aims of devolution and the New Federalism has been noted by Smith and Sosin (2001):

> Proponents of faith-based agencies are a diverse lot. Some simply hope that faith-based agencies are more effective than traditional public and nonprofit service delivery. Others hope that faith-based agencies *will reduce demands on the state*, promote a greater role for faith in public life, and in the long run, *shrink the state by shifting responsibility for social problems to faith-based agencies, churches, and local communities.* (page 30, italics added)

Whether governmental support of faith-based programs is generally seen as the sincere expression of the religious views of political leaders, or as cynical and hypocritical, depends upon one's political orientation. What is clear is that the outcomes of such restructuring on a tremendous scale remain to be seen, as to date these outsourcing-privatizing-downsizing and faith-based initiatives have been a governmental policy shaped largely by faith, philosophy, ideology, and hoped-for cost savings, not by empirical data. For example, the Governor of Florida, Jeb Bush, (himself a devout Roman Catholic, and the President's brother), recently established a unique state prison, aimed at housing prisoners of faith (Christian, Jew, Muslim, etc.) and providing faith-based counseling services to assist in their rehabilitation. The faith-based prison regimen is less rigorous than that prevailing in the more common secular prisons within the state, in return for exemplary behavior on the part of the prisoners. One looked-for outcome of this new faith-based prison is a greatly reduced recidivism rate among its discharged prisoners, relative to that obtained from those who serve their time in conventional prisons.

But there are some points of light, to plagiarize a phrase, for the secularly-oriented, empirically-based social service professional to take some comfort in, and these consist of the oft-reiterated assertion by Federal officials that faith-based social service programs are to be funded because of their *effectiveness*, not their religious orientation. For example:

> . . . when we make decisions on public funding, we should not focus on the religion you practice, *but on the results you deliver*. (President George W. Bush, 29 October 2003, italics added, *www. whitehouse.gov/news/releases/2003/10/20031029-10.html*),

> The paramount goal is compassionate results . . . to ensure that the efforts of faith-based and other community organizations meet high standards of excellence and accountability. (Executive Order, 29 January 2001, *www.whitehouse.gov/news/releases/2001/01/ 20010129-2.html*)

> . . . President Bush wants the federal government to partner with the best provider of social services–secular or sacred. And in the competition for these dollars, he wants to end discrimination against faith-based groups. For years, these groups were either prohibited from applying or discouraged from applying to provide public services. It isn't about funding religion–President Bush does not want government to fund religion. It is about getting results: addicts in recovery, the homeless off the street and into stable lives, and the children of prisoners in mentoring programs where they are loved and educated. (Ask the White House. 22 June 2004. Interview with Jim Towey, *www.whitehouse.gov/ask/20040622. html*)

The creation of various typologies to categorize faith-based organizations has been undertaken by a number of writers (e.g., Jeavons, 1998; Smith & Sosin, 2001; Unruh & Sider, 205), but these analyze agencies along different dimensions, such as denominational affiliation, degree of secular vs. religious financial support, extent of secular service provision, etc. This is in truth, an arcane topic. Without attempting to replicate such efforts, in the author's view for the purposes of contemplating a program evaluation, faith-based programs can be approximately categorized into three types:

Type 1–Those Staffed or Financially Supported by Persons of Faith, Who Provide Solely Secular Services

Some examples might be church groups who support with finances, supplies, and staff, a local soup kitchen or homeless shelter; services provided by members of the Church of Jesus Christ of Latter-Day Saints (LDS), such as free food, clothing, tsunami relief, or job counseling to non-church members, absent any proselytizing (see Rudd, 1995, for a marvelous exposition of the impressive national and international LDS church welfare programs); health care provided by a hospital supported by a Roman Catholic order of nuns, etc. In these programs the services are obviously material and secular, and intended primarily to improve the material and secular circumstances of peoples' lives. These programs are very amenable to scientific investigations of outcomes, as both the independent variable (intervention program) and dependent variables (outcomes), are measurable and observable.

Type 2–Those Staffed by Persons of Faith Who Provide Services Which Contain an Element of Religious Teaching or Practice as a Provision of Service Itself, and Which Is Intended to Produce Some Demonstrable, Observable Effects

Examples here include membership in Alcoholics Anonymous, wherein the 12-Step Program contains some formal and explicit steps designed to produce a spiritual awakening, leading to abstinence from alcohol; The Boys Scouts of America, whose oath includes pledging one's duty to God, and the ability to earn various religious awards, and whose Scout troops contain an officer called the Chaplain. But much of the Scouting program seems on the surface very secular, and the non-theist is generally able to participate without hindrance, hypocrisy or discomfort; intercessory prayer, focused on producing a physical healing of an ill individual, or to bring peace to a distressed person or family; wearing a Kabbalah Red String for protection; or group transcendental meditation aimed at reducing crime. An early example would be the supposed miracle of the Gadarene Swine, as recounted in the Book of Luke in the New Testament–Jesus was visiting the land of the Gadarenes, and came across a man possessed by numerous demons. Jesus commanded the demons to leave him, which they did, entering instead into a herd of nearby swine who fled into a lake and drowned. In these programs the intervention is at least in part faith-based, but the presumptive effects should be evident in the physical world in which we live. Such programs can lend themselves to empirical evaluations of outcome, even though the independent variable (intervention) is difficult, if not impossible, to operationalize.

Type 3–Those Staffed by Persons of Faith Who Provide Solely Religious Services, Intended to Produce Supernatural Changes

Such programs are not so much social service programs as evangelical ones, primarily aimed at bringing about a religious conversion, e.g., become saved, as opposed to changing the material circumstances of a person's life. The intervention is invisible, and the purported effects are similarly transcendental. A newly 'saved' person may look and act outwardly the same, but the inward spiritual transformation is said to be a profound and permanent one. These programs would not seem to lend themselves to any form of scientific evaluation inasmuch as they purportedly yield *supernatural* changes, not ones occurring or evident in the natural world in which we live, and in that the intervention itself is immaterial. Science can take no position regarding the validity of such supernatural claims, inasmuch as its purview is the physical, natural world.

It would also seem evident that the first type of faith-based program listed above would easily meet constitutional standards permitting it to receive Federal funding to deliver social services, and the second type as well, in limited circumstances. The third type would seem to be precluded from receiving any form of payment from taxpayers. This categorization scheme begins to provide the social worker with some points of leverage in regard to evaluating faith-based programs.

Elsewhere (Thyer, 2001, pp. 17-18) I have described several axioms about measurement and treatment which have some bearing on the topic of evidence-based practice and faith-based programs:

Axiom 1: If something exists, then it has the potential to be measured.

Axiom 2: If something can be measured, then the practitioner is in a better position to do something about it.

Axiom 3: If a client problem can be validly measured, then the social worker is in a better position to effectively help the client and to see whether the efforts are followed by improvements in the client's life.

The capacity to be able to describe some anticipated *outcome* of a faith-based program is the key point of leverage of beginning to apply scientific principles of evaluation to that program. If this outcome can be cast into the language of one or more operationally defined, reliable and valid approach to *measuring* said outcomes, then the stage is set to embark upon the design of a suitable evaluation strategy. The reader will note that I did not state that one needs to have a replicable *intervention* in order to conduct a program evaluation. This is a deliberate omission, and I have provided a rationale for it elsewhere:

Myth #4–You Must Only Study Extremely Well Proceduralized Interventions

> Clear specification of the 'independent variable' is indeed characteristic of conventional social and behavioral science research. But social work practice largely lacks this element. Child protective services, school social work, domestic violence work, community organizing, all are difficult to proceduralize. If one accepts the myth that you need to have a well-proceduralized intervention, then you will be discouraged from doing evaluation research. We social workers are different from conventional social and behavioral scientists–our 'independent variable' or treatment programs, are NOT well described. But this should not deter us from trying to evaluate their outcomes. (Thyer, 2002, p. 12, bold in original)

If a practitioner can measure client outcomes at some point after receipt of a faith-based program, and can do this for a number (ideally everyone who received the program, or at least a genuinely representative sample of them) of such clients, then the potential exists to conduct a one-group post-treatment only study, diagrammed as X-O, with X representing the service, and O representing an assessment. For example, one measure of the effectiveness of Florida's new faith-based prison would be to assess recidivism of its released prisons, at some meaningful period of time after release, say two years later. If say, zero percent of the prisoners had been reincarcerated, one would be inclined to rate the faith-based prison a success, perhaps justifying the expenditure of taxpayers money on a faith-based program. If 95 percent had been reincarcerated, then it would likely be deemed a failure, and consideration should be given to discontinuing the prison. Generally speaking, exceptionally clear and compelling results *do not* require extensive control groups or complicated statistical analysis. These latter features of program evaluation design are only needed when the effects of the intervention are highly variable or modest in their influence.

This then is the intersection of how empirically-oriented (if not also faith-based) social researchers can helpfully collaborate with faith-based social service programs–*in the design and conduct of program evaluation studies intended to help determine whether or not these programs are achieving their intended goals.* Virtually *any* faith-based program that is intended to produce observable results in the physical, material world in which clients live, (which, as it happens, forms the majority of the issues which social service professionals are called upon to address), is potentially amenable to scientific investigation of its empirical outcomes. In the preliminary stages of program evaluation, it really does not matter exactly how *Alcoholics Anonymous* really works, or if the spiritual aspects of that widespread program are an essential component to treatment success. One simply needs to be able to ascertain *outcomes*. Once it has been convincingly shown that a given program does indeed produce reliably effective results, *then* it may be worthwhile to undertake process studies, or componential analyses of the intervention's critical ingredients. Given that many, if not most, potential social programs will *not*, in the fullness of time, be shown to be effective, it makes sense to hold off on studies of process until one is sure that the treatment itself is truly useful.

In general, program evaluations could profitably be designed to address the following types of questions, in the order given:

1. Do clients receiving the program get initially better?
2. Do clients receiving the program demonstrate greater initial improvements, relative to those who did not receive the program?
3. Do clients receiving the program demonstrate greater initial improvements, relative to those receiving placebo or sham treatment?

4. Do clients receiving the program demonstrate greater initial improvements, relative to those receiving standard care?

If the answers to the above questions are positive, then more complex inquiries may be warranted, as in:

5. Do the positive results endure for a long time?
6. Is the intervention effective across a diverse array of clients?
7. Is the intervention effective when applied in everyday practice settings?

Each of these sequential questions requires an increasingly sophisticated research design (and time, money and other resources) to be effectively answered, hence the recommendation to address the earlier ones first. Fortunately, relatively simple and inexpensive research methods *can be used* to answer the first question, as in the example given of evaluating the faith-based prison described above.

Some years ago, the author was involved in a program evaluation of a homeless shelter, whose associate director was completing his masters degree, and who sought some help from the author in evaluating the program's services. The graduate student was very much a devoted Christian, and he chose social services as his career so that he could apply his faith. Moreover he elected to work with homeless persons as among the most destitute of persons. The homeless shelter's services were exclusively secular–shelter, meals, clothing, job placement, and assistance in finding safe, long term and affordable housing. One significant measure of its success would be the proportion of formerly served clients who, some time after their receipt of shelter assistance in finding a home, were still residing in acceptable housing circumstances. The student chose a four month time period during the previous year, and divided all clients (head-of-household) served during that time into transient persons seeking assistance (n = 24), versus those with a long term history of living in the local community (n = 100). Through vigorous efforts, follow-up contact was made over a three week period with 71 (71%) of these 100 heads-of-houses served last year at the homeless shelter, with a history of living in the local community. The average follow-up period was 38 weeks after leaving the homeless shelter. It was found that 58% of the clients held leases/rental agreements (reflective of relatively stable housing), and had lived there an average of 18 weeks. Most residents rated their homes as a relatively 'safe' place in which to live. This evaluation project ultimately resulted in a publication (Glisson, Thyer & Fischer, 2001) one of the very few ever published which empirically examined the extent to which discharged homeless shelter clients remained in safe and stable housing. The favorable results were gratefully received by the shelter's board of directors, and were used in future fund-raising efforts. In terms of a research design, this could be conceived of as a one-group posttest-only design, and diagrammed as simply an X-O design, with X being the intervention, and O being the status of the clients at follow-up.

Layer, Roberts, Wild and Walters (2004) evaluated the effectiveness of a spiritual group intervention derived from a Christian tradition, with 35 women who experienced post-abortion grief (PAG). The women were assessed in terms of shame and trauma symptoms before group work, and again immediately after the semi-structured group work intervention, finding significant improvements following the intervention. The writers' keen religious convictions are evident throughout the writing of this report, and its publication in a mainstream social research journal again exemplifies the synergistic results which can be brought about through a judicious integration of faith-based services and empirically-oriented program evaluation methods. This design could be graphed as an O-X-O design, with pretest assessments occurring before participation in post-abortion grief group work, and again after group work.

A more complex evaluation of a faith-based program was reported by Wolf and Abell (2003). David Wolf was a doctoral student in social work at Florida State University, and a practitioner of a form of Hindu-derived meditation methods. For his dissertation Wolf conducted a randomized controlled study, assigning clients seeking help for stress and depression to one of three groups. The treatment group received instruction in, and practiced, 'real' meditation (involving the repetition of a legitimate form of meditative chanting), the placebo group receiving instruction and practice in sham chanting meditation methods, and the no-treatment group receiving nothing. Each group consisted of 31 participants. Assessments of stress and depression were made at the beginning of the program, again after four weeks of 'treatment' for the first two groups, and again, four weeks after meditation instruction was halted. It was found that the group receiving 'real' meditation training improved more than the clients receiving sham meditation instruction, or the non-treatment group. While there are many more details to this study, it does represent a nice approach to empirically evaluate the effectiveness of one approach to prayer which claims to reduce stress and depression, an approach which appeared to support this particular faith-based program. Schematically, this design looks like this:

```
R   O   X   O   O
R   O   Y   O   O
R   O       O   O
```

with R indicating that each group was created via random assignment, X being exposure to 'real' meditation methods, Y being provided 'sham' meditation methods, and the third group receiving no meditation instruction at all.

> This study is also a nice example of the scenario described by Bruno so many years ago:
>
> The inclusion of projects of social work among the activities of religious bodies affords ample opportunity for the demonstration of any unique or superior quality inherent in such a controlling philosophy. (Bruno, 1936, p. 398)

In other words, if a faith-based program is superior to alternative methods of providing social intervention, a suitably controlled experimental study is a very strong method to demonstrate this.

A more ambitious prospectively designed study of the effects of religious meditation was undertaken during the summer of 1993, when almost 4000 practitioners of transcendental meditation gathered for an 8 week period in Washington, DC. Their purpose was to purposively meditate, in order to test the hypothesis that large numbers of meditators could reduce violent crime in the District of Columbia. Here the independent variable was a faith-based intervention, Hindu meditation, and the dependent variable was government-collected statistics on crime. The research design involved the technique called time-series anlysis. Reportedly, violence crime decreased by 23%, a statistically significant result, during the 8 weeks of purposive meditation (see Hagelin et al., 1999)! This interesting work appeared in a quality peer-reviewed journal, and further illustrates how faith-based programs can be amenable to scientific investigation as to outcomes.

Conducting a program evaluation assumes a commitment to properly using scientific methodology, and to accepting the results of a properly conducted study, regardless of one's personal investment in a program.

Sometimes the results of an empirical study *do not* support the effectiveness of a given social intervention, be it faith-based or not. An example of this was the well-designed study by Aviles et al. (2001) in evaluating the efficacy of intercessory prayer. This was a randomized controlled, and double-blind study to test the hypothesis that intercessory prayer could improve the health outcomes of patients on a cardiac treatment unit. Prayer was found to have no effects at all. It requires real moral integrity for a researcher to commit to publishing such negative results. I hasten to add that my citing the above two studies are not an endorsement of their findings, only of my admiration for the authors' ambition and willingness to undertake a program evaluation. Empirical research on the effectiveness of faith-based interventions *is* an imminently do-able undertaking for social researchers, and when public monies are devoted to the provision of such services, the ethical mandate to rigorously evaluate the results is heightened.

One caveat here–*The effectiveness of a faith-based program in no way validates the theology underlying the program.* Healing via the laying on of hands is a part of many disparate religious traditions, Christian, Jewish, Hindu, Muslim, etc. The presumptive mechanisms of action, the theological theory, if you will, is considerably different among these traditions. The Christian will likely ascribe any miraculous healing results to the healer being a channel for either Jesus or the Holy Spirit, while the Hindu priest who obtains similarly 'miraculous' results would claim to have channeled pranic energy, or perhaps was visited by Sri Ramakrishna, in effecting a cure. Theologically *both* healers can't be right. In a more secular example, it may turn out that the cognitive-behavioral psychotherapy called eye-movement desensitization and reprocessing (EMDR) therapy can help clients with certain mental health problems, but it has long been established that the theoretical mechanisms originally proposed to account for the presumptive success of EMDR are incorrect (Van Deusen, 2004). The providers of faith-based program need not shrink from subjecting the results of their services to scientific analysis, given the disconnect between empirical outcomes, and the potential validity or invalidity of underlying theory or theology. The material successes of a faith-based program do not reflect the validity of the principles of faith that program is derived from. Science is not in the business of attempting to refute or validate anyone's theological beliefs (e.g., "Is God a triune being?"), belonging as these do to the realm of the supernatural, and are impervious to empirical analysis.

CONCLUSION

After some decades of being subject to neglect or contempt, faith-based social care programs are receiving increased attention and resources enabling them to undertake a greater role in the national network of human services. Faith-based programs receiving public support can expect to be rightly scrutinized by the public, in terms of their ability to attain professed program goals. The tools of conventional empirically-oriented program evaluation research have tremendous potential to help demonstrate the effectiveness of faith-based programs, which will justify their ongoing support from public funds. Negative research findings can be properly scrutinized by the faith-based community of service providers to help make tough, data-based, decisions on funding priorities. Several examples are described, illustrating how various types of faith-based programs have profitably participated in program evaluation studies.

REFERENCES

Abbot, G. (1931). *Social welfare and professional education.* Chicago: University of Chicago Press.

Aviles, J. M., Whelan, E., & Hernke, D.A. et al. (2001). Intercessory prayer and cardiovascular disease progression in a coronary care population: A randomized controlled trial. *Mayo Clinic Proceedings, 76,* 1192-1198.

Barker, R. (Ed.). (2003). *The social work dictionary* (5th edition). Washington, DC: NASW Press.

Belcher, J. R., Fandetti, D., & Cole, D. (2004). Is Christian religious conservatism compatible with the liberal social welfare state? *Social Work, 49,* 269-276.

Bruno, F. A. (1936). *The theory of social work.* New York: D. C. Health.

Chaiklin, H. (2005). Franklin Benjamin Sanborn: Human services innovator. *Research on Social Work Practice, 15,* 127-134.

Cheney, A. (1926). *The nature and scope of social work.* New York: American Association of Social Workers.

Comte, A. (1853). *The positive philosophy.* New York: Calvin Blanchard.

Garland, D. R. (1995). Church social work. In R. L. Edwards (Ed.). *Encyclopedia of social work* (19th edition, pp. 475-483). Washington, DC: National Association of Social Workers.

Glisson, G. M., Thyer, B. A., & Fischer, R. L. (2001). Serving the homeless: Evaluating the effectiveness of homeless shelter services. *Journal of Sociology and Social Welfare, 28*(4), 89-97.

Hagelin, J. S., Rainforth, M. V., Cavanaugh, K. L., Alexander, C. N., Shatkin, S. F., Davies, J. L., Hughes, A. O., Ross, E., & Orme-Johnson, D. W. (1999). Effects of group practice of the transcendental meditation program on preventing violent crime in Washington, DC: Results of the National Demonstration Project, June-July 93. *Social Indicators Research, 47*(2), 153-201.

Hamilton, G. (1940). *Theory and practice of social casework.* New York: Columbia University Press.

Harp, G. J. (1995). *Positivist republic: Auguste Comte and the reconstruction of American liberalism, 1865-1920.* University Park, PA: Pennsylvania State University Press.

Haskell, T. L. (2000). *The emergence of professional social science: The American Social Science Association and the nineteenth century crisis of authority.* Baltimore, MD: Johns Hopkins University Press.

Hawkins, R. L. *Auguste Comte and the United States 1816-1853.* Cambridge, MA: Harvard University Press.

Hodge, D. (2002). Does social work oppress evangelical Christians? A 'new class' analysis of society and social work. *Social Work, 47,* 401-414.

Jeavons, T. (1998). Identifying characteristics of 'relious' organizations: An exploratory proposal. In N. J. Demerath, P. D. Hall, T. Schmit, & R. W. Williams (Eds.). *Sacred companies: Organizational aspects of religious and religious aspects of organizations* (pp. 79-96). New York: Oxford University Press.

Johnson, F. E. (1941). Protestant social work. In R. H. Kurtz (Ed.). *Social work year book* (pp. 403-412). New York: Russell Sage Foundation.

Layer, S. D., Roberts, C., Wild, K., & Walters, J. (2004). Post-abortion grief: Evaluating the possible efficacy of a spiritual group intervention. *Research on Social Work Practice, 14,* 344-350.

Lubov, R (1972). *The professional altruist: The emergence of social work as a career 1880-1930.* New York: Atheneum.

Mill, J. S. (1887). *The positive philosophy of Auguste Comte.* Honolulu, HI: University Press of the Pacific (reprinted in 2002).

Pickering, M. (1995). *Auguste Comte: An intellectual biography.* New York: Cambridge University Press.

Queen, S. A. (1927). Contrasted approaches to social problems. *Proceedings, Seventh National Conference on Social Service of the Protestant Episcopal Church.*

Reynolds, B. C. (1942). *Learning and teaching in the practice of social work.* New York: Farrar & Rinehart.

Richmond, M. (1890). Our relation to the churches. In M. Richmond (1930). *The long view* (pp. 115-119). New York: Russell Sage Foundation.

Richmond, M. (1917). *Social diagnosis.* New York: Russell Sage Foundation.

Rudd, G. L. (1995). *Pure religion: The story of church welfare services since 1930.* Salt Lake City, UT: The Church of Jesus Christ of Latter-Day Saints.

Sanzenbach, P. (1989). Religion and social work: It's not that simple. *Journal for the Scientific Study of Religion, 70,* 571-572.

Smith, S. R., & Sosin, M. R. (2001). The varieties of faith-related agencies. *Public Aministration Review, 61,* 651-699.

Thyer, B. A. (Ed.) (2001). *Handbook of social work research methods.* Thousand Oaks, CA: Sage.

Thyer, B. A. (2002). Evaluation of social work practice in the new millennium: Myths and realities. In D. T. L. Shek, L. M. Chow, A. C. Fai, & J. J. Lee (Eds.). *Advances in social welfare in Hong Kong* (pp. 3-18). Hong Kong: The Chinese University of Hong Kong

Thyer, B. A. (2004). Science and evidence-based social work practice. In H. E. Briggs & T. L. Rzepnicki (Eds.). *Using evidence in social work practice* (pp. 74-89). Chicago, IL: Lyceum Books.

Todd, A. J. (1920). *The scientific spirit and social work*. New York: Macmillan.

Unruh, H. R., & Sider, R. J. (2005). *Saving souls, serving society: Understanding the faith factor in church-based social ministry*. New York: Oxford University Press.

Van Deusen, K. M. (2004). Bilateral stimulation in EMDR: A replicated single-subject component analysis. *Behavior Therapist, 27*(4), 79-86.

Warner, A. G. (1908). *American charities (revised edition)*. New York: Thomas Y. Crowell.

Warner, A. G., Queen, S. A., & Harper, E. B. (1930). *American charities and social work*. New York: Thomas Y. Crowell.

Wolf, D. B., & Abell, N. (2003). Examining the effects of meditation techniques on psychosocial functioning. *Research on Social Work Practice, 13,* 27-42.

Chapter 5

Social Service Research and Religion: Thoughts About How to Measure Intervention-Based Impact

David A. Zanis
Ram A. Cnaan

SUMMARY. Development of accountability standards to demonstrate cause and effect relationships are gaining rapid advancement in the field of social sciences. Many governmental agencies, foundations, and other

David A. Zanis, PhD, is Associate Professor in the School of Social Administration at Temple University. He is the founder of Clinical Outcomes Group, a non-profit health and social service program in Central Pennsylvania. Dr. Zanis has published in the areas of substance abuse treatment effectiveness and program evaluation.

Ram A. Cnaan, PhD, is Professor and Director of the Program for Religion and Social Policy Research at the University of Pennsylvania, School of Social Policy & Practice. He has published widely in the areas of religion and social care and community practice. He is the author of: *The Newer Deal: Social Work and Religion in Partnership* (Columbia University Press, 1999), *The Invisible Caring Hand: American Congregations and the Provision of Welfare* (New York University Press, 2002), and *The Other Philadelphia Story: How Local Congregations Support Quality of Life in Urban America* (University of Pennsylvania Press, 2006).

Address correspondence to: Ram A. Cnaan, PhD, School of Social Policy and Practice, University of Pennsylvania, 3701 Locust Walk, Philadelphia, PA 19104 (E-mail: cnaan@ssw.upenn.edu).

[Haworth co-indexing entry note]: "Social Service Research and Religion: Thoughts About How to Measure Intervention-Based Impact." Zanis, David A., and Ram A. Cnaan. Co-published simultaneously in *Journal of Religion & Spirituality in Social Work* (The Haworth Pastoral Press, an imprint of The Haworth Press, Inc.) Vol. 25, No. 3/4, 2006, pp. 83-104; and: *Faith-Based Social Services: Measures, Assessments, and Effectiveness* (ed: Stephanie C. Boddie, and Ram A. Cnaan) The Haworth Pastoral Press, an imprint of The Haworth Press, Inc., 2006, pp. 83-104.

funders have developed approaches that require organizations to utilize science-based programs and incorporate evaluative methods to show improved outcomes and cost benefits to society. This article will examine the need for increased accountability in developing effective interventions by faith-based organizations in the delivery of social service interventions. Recently, there has been a strong movement toward governmental funding for faith-based institutions to provide social services, although there has been inadequate scientific data to demonstrate that approaches implemented are effective in meeting needs or yielding favorable outcomes. Similarly, many faith-based organizations provide innovative and effective programs that could serve as model programs if there was appropriate empirical evidence. This article will discuss how rigorous evaluative approaches such as randomized clinical control trials can produce scientific data on program effectiveness. We will use a case example in the field of drug and alcohol treatment to illustrate these points.

KEYWORDS. Faith-based intervention, cost-effectiveness, control clinical trials, social services, substance abuse

Contrary to expectations in what otherwise has become an age of science and empirical evidence, most Americans did not turn secular, and religion occupies an important role in their lives. In the fields of education and scientific inquiry, however, empirical scientists dominate and medical and social sciences have both opposed and resisted the inclusion of the religious issues in research (Cnaan, Wineburg, & Boddie, 1999). However, we are also living in an era in which politicians, and especially the Clinton and Bush administrations, are harnessing faith-based providers to assist in the education and social service delivery fields. Such inclusion of new actors cannot go unevaluated.

How can we promote partnership between public resources and faith-based service provision if we do not follow it with careful evaluation? There is ample anecdotal information to praise faith-based providers for their successful and heroic work. However, there are no conclusive scientific studies demonstrating the effectiveness of faith based interventions using the most rigorous scientific methods. Johnson (2002) reviewed some 800 studies that claim to have covered faith-based social interventions and found that only 25 of them attempted to provide any form of intervention evaluation and even these did not use rigorous methodologies. The lack of empirical evidence creates skepticism by the scientific community and has limited opportunities for advancement in understanding how faith based programs can be fully integrated within a systematic framework of social service delivery.

To assess the impact of faith-based social programs, social scientists are obliged to harness the most rigorous evaluation methods, Randomized Control Clinical Trials (RCCT), to determine the relative contributions of faith-based social interventions. Assessing the capacity of a program to produce a cause and effect relationship is an incremental process and involves several stages including: (1) Does the proposed intervention cause the participants in the program to improve? (2) To what degree do the participants in the program improve compared to other valid interventions? (3) Can the program be replicated in other communities? (4) Is the program cost-beneficial to society compared to other valid approaches? These stages will be illustrated and described.

RANDOMIZED CLINICAL CONTROLLED TRIALS (RCCTS)

Randomized clinical controlled trial (RCCT) was originated in biomedical research and has been increasingly applied in field experiments in social program evaluation. The role of RCCTs is to enable the researcher to control for threats to the internal and external validity or the possibility of alternative explanatory factors of the studied intervention. In this article, only the basic experimental design is presented and the ways it deals with possible threats to yield valid conclusions.

The natural and behavioral sciences have long used a quasi-experimental approach to research. Unlike laboratory experiments, these experiments are conducted in naturalistic contexts (Boruch, 1997; Orr, 1999) such as clinics, welfare agencies, schools, etc. The advantage of this type of experiment is that findings are more realistic and can be generalized. The disadvantage is that the non-laboratory setting makes it more difficult to control for confounding variables. In this context, the RCCT, although costly in terms of time and money, is important because its design makes it possible to control for biases that may affect the validity and generalizability of the study.

The basic experimental design is a field experiment that has a treatment group and a control group. Unlike other group comparisons such as quasi-experiments, the experimental design: (1) compares those receiving an experimental treatment (treatment group) with those receiving standard treatment or an alternate treatment (comparison group) or no treatment (control group), (2) randomly assigns participants to either the treatment or control/comparison group, and (3) takes relevant outcome measurements of both groups following the completion of treatment. Failure to include all three steps may invalidate results. Lack of one or more of those steps does not necessarily render the study improper, but confounds the ability to validate the results and introduces bias.

Bias is defined as systematic error introduced into sampling or testing that influences outcome. In general terms, validity refers to the extent to which the conclusions about the effects of the intervention are well founded and can be further generalized to other populations or communities. In the following section, the key threats to validity that may invalidate results and the ways in which the RCCT attempts to control for them are discussed.

Internal Validity

Internal validity is concerned with the demonstrated correlation and presumed causality between the intervention and the changes observed (Allison, 1995; Brinberg & McGrath, 1985; Campbell, 1969; Campbell & Stanley, 1963; Cook & Campbell, 1979; Greenhouse, Stangl & Bromberg, 1989). These threats, which may interact with one another, are known as: (1) history, (2) maturation, (3) testing, (4) statistical regression to the mean, (5) selection bias or participants, (6) attrition and experimental mortality, (7) lack of protocol compliance, (8) instrumentation error, and (9) participant crossover. Each of these 9 threats to internal validity could serve as a possible explanation for change unless measures are undertaken to negate their influence.

To control for these threats to internal validity, important steps must be taken in the experimental design. (a) The first of these is the use of random assignment to the control and experimental groups which enables the researchers to minimize the threat emanating from possible biases such as history, testing, regression towards the mean, and selection. Randomized assignment creates an "equal chance" for each individual to belong to either of the groups. (b) The combination of this design with process evaluation or "monitoring," using qualitative methods and in-depth interviews, can further help rule out alternative explanations to the results. It can also help identify possible new hypotheses that may lead to further research. Importantly, the intervention must be delivered as proposed so that a cause and effect relationship can be evaluated. (c) The use of advanced statistical procedures, such as event-history analysis, can minimize biases arising from attrition and history. (d) Implementation of suitable incentives and controls, such as material incentives and explanation of the importance of the study and its design, will minimize crossover and attrition problems that may jeopardize the study. Precautions should also be taken with regard to the staff of the program so that they do not influence or impact one another or the clients across groups.

External Validity

External validity relates to the degree to which the results can be generalized beyond the study population to the general population. Threats that may compromise the generalizability of evaluation experiments have been widely discussed in the literature (Bracht & Glass, 1968; Brinberg & McGrath, 1985; Cook & Campbell, 1979; Campbell & Stanley, 1963; Kazdin, 1992). These threats, which may again interact with one another, are known as: characteristics of the sample, stimulus characteristics, reactivity of experimental arrangements, reactivity of assessment, contamination, multiple treatment interference, test sensitization, novelty/Hawthorne effects, and time-effects.

To control for external threats that can invalidate the generalizability of the findings, two important steps are required. First, the experiment should be replicated in different contexts of time, sites, and clients. Basing a new intervention policy on one well crafted study is dangerous as results can be biased by the unique characteristics of the specific study (Brody, 1998). In the behavioral and social sciences, however, it is imperative to use multiple trials and comparisons to substantiate a claim for definitive and generalizable results (Campbell & Rouso, 1999). Second, the design of the intervention must provide for ongoing monitoring and process evaluation, using in-depth interviews and systematic observation whenever possible (Rossi, Freeman, & Lipsey, 1999). This will enable the researchers to: (a) ascertain that the intervention was carried out according to the intervention protocol, and that randomization was not compromised; and (b) assess the reactions of the clients to the intervention, the setting, and the clinicians or professionals involved.

DEVELOPMENT OF AN INTERVENTION APPROACH

Design Lessons from Biomedical

Importantly any proposed intervention undergoes a variety of preliminary steps on standardizing the intervention approach prior to investing valuable resources on conducting an experimental design. For example, Zanis (2005) reported that the stages of intervention developmental work and pilot testing prior to an experimental design took approximately 10 years to refine. This developmental work includes refining the intervention to determine several factors including: (1) the theoretical approach, (2) the actual content of the intervention; (3) the amount of time necessary to delivery the intervention; (4) the approach of the intervention; and (5) a basic understanding on how participants respond to the delivery of the intervention.

Many faith-based organizations have a general idea that their program is effective and the program produces positive outcomes. Positive outcomes are often discovered in two general ways. First, the outcomes are often intended, meaning that the organization developed a hypothesis and designed a specific intervention to yield an expected outcome. Secondly, an intervention approach could be developed based on an unintended outcome, meaning that a favorable outcome was observed although it was not anticipated. Regardless of how the intervention was discovered, the purported outcomes of the intervention must be measured by valid instruments and methods to determine that a cause and effect relationship exists. The intervention (cause) is then tested in an incremental approach to determine if the effects are valid and other potential rival hypotheses could be ruled out as causal determinants. Thus, the ideas for new interventions and clinical trials are often based on what organizations have implemented in practice.

The research design that best minimizes these potential threats is the RCCT. The RCCT format developed for biomedical research may be categorized by four phases. A Phase-1 trial is generally performed when a new treatment method is proposed. The sample size is limited and the frequency of data collection per person is high. The purpose is to detect any negative or side effects to the treatment that might occur over short-term use. Typically, this phase requires about 20 subjects.

A Phase-2 trial involves a larger sample (20-100 subjects). The purpose is to provide preliminary information regarding the efficacy of the new treatment versus other modes of treatment. Phase-2 studies are used to identify therapies that should be tested in a large-scale clinical trial and eliminate the widespread use of ineffective interventions.

A Phase-3 trial, often the final and largest phase, compares the new treatment with the standard treatment, other experimental treatments, or a no-treatment option to determine its efficacy among certain subgroups. For example, does the proposed intervention produce a similar effect for individuals regardless of age, income, and other possible demographic interactions? The sample size is usually large (several hundred subjects), and the sample size is calculated using statistical formulas so that chance findings are ruled out.

A Phase-4 trial is used to follow-up the long-term effects (usually beyond a one-year period) and safety of a treatment that successfully passed the previous phases and has been approved for public use (Meinert & Tonascia, 1986).

The basic characteristics of any randomized controlled clinical trial are the following: (a) it is carried out on human beings who provide voluntary consent to participate in a research study, (b) it is designed to assess the effectiveness of one or more modes of intervention by examining possible changes in participant knowledge, opinion, attitude, motivation, behaviors, etc., (c) it is preceded by the preparation of a very detailed protocol, that includes a step-by step guide on the delivery of the intervention and standardized training of personnel involved in the delivery of services. Also monitoring of service delivery through audiotapes, videotapes, or direct observation; (d) clients are randomly selected for one of the relevant study groups, (e) if possible, blind treatment is provided, (f) in order to accrue a large enough number of subjects, it is done preferably in a multi-center arrangement, (g) pre-treatment data are carefully selected and collected for each client for as long as possible, and the use of collateral data to measure outcomes is highly desirable (e.g., treatment records), and (h) response data are collected in a systematic timeline for as long as the study is under way.

Conducting a RCCT is an incremental, tedious, and expensive endeavor, enabling the researchers to control for potential threats that may be involved in evaluating program efficacy and efficiency, while requiring an investment in terms of time, human and fiscal resources. The major justification for such endeavor is the immense potential it holds for substantiating the effectiveness and efficacy of social interventions for broader implementation and replication.

Examining Design Factors Associated with the Development of Faith-Based Interventions

As noted by Johnson (2002) there have been dozens of faith-based approaches published in the scientific literature. However, few of these studies have developed and defined the exact elements of what the intervention approach consists. Koenig, McCullough, and Larson (2001) operationalized the basic differences between religion and spirituality. Religion is an organized system of beliefs, practices, rituals and symbols designed to: (1) facilitate closeness to the sacred or a transcendent higher power, and (2) foster an understanding of a person's relationship and responsibility to others in living together in a community. Whereas Spirituality is defined as the personal quest for understanding answers to ultimate questions about life, meaning and about relationship to a higher power which may lead to the development of participation in a religion. Given, these broad definitions, a clear understanding on how religion and or spirituality is operationalized and delivered within a faith-based intervention is necessary in order for the approach to be compared to other valid intervention approaches.

The fields of religion studies and faith-based social service have been guided historically by practices based in personal and professional belief systems. By using RCCT, we are presented with the potential to establish the effectiveness of interventions. This opportunity defines the subtle division between practice as art and practice as science. The experimental design creates the bridge between personal and professional beliefs and the actual reality of outcomes, between theory-based practice and its impact. Many people hope that faith-based social interventions will fail or succeed each based on their set of beliefs; however, only rigorous research designs such as RCCTs can provide appropriate information to further practice and policy development. One specific field where RCCT's potential can be demonstrated is faith-based substance abuse rehabilitation.

The Relationship Between Faith Based Interventions and Substance Abuse

The etiology of substance abuse is inconclusive. It is widely agreed, however, that a successful recovery, one that lasts for a significant period of time, includes some form of personal transformation and change in life style. Yet, rates of successful recovery are low and many abusers turn back to use their substance of choice. It is worth considering the claim that the likelihood of a successful recovery may be raised for some substance abusers through careful use of spirituality, religion, and organized religion (Miller, 1990; 1997). Some individuals, if they are offered a bridge to their spirituality and a sense of religiosity may find a renewed strength for continued improvements in both abstinence from substances and change in their quality of life. This is clearly not true for each and every person with an addiction, but then no single method of intervention is effective for everyone. Religion and spirituality are said to enable the individual to acknowledge his/her lack of control and thereby paradoxically use it to gain more control over the habit of using addictive substances. The importance of addictive substances in one's life may be reduced by the recognition that a higher being exists and that one needs to find a path toward this being and act appropriately (Miller et al., 1997; Gorsuch, 1995). Furthermore, becoming a member of a local religious congregation could make it easier to develop a positive peer support system in place of social isolation, family and friends who are a negative influence and do not understand recovery. Congregational members are capable of providing moral guidance and support, setting healthy standards, supporting the individual with tangible tasks, spending time with the recovering individual through socializing in non-substance related activities, and forming a group of emotional support. Consequently, the person in recovery may try not to disappoint the congregational members and will work harder to maintain abstinence. In other words, congregational-based group dynamics coupled with pro-social values of religion, and one's personal spiritual reflections, may create a process most conducive for substance recovery. One theoretical approach that could guide studies in this area is a combination of adopting a spiritual understanding (e.g., positive power of meaning of life) and or engagement in a religion (Koenig, McCullough, and Larson, 2001).

The empirical data on the role of religion in helping people abstain from drugs and alcohol are limited and methodologically weak. Reviewing the addiction literature shows few instances of randomized experiments and almost no use of RCCT. It is this lack of convincing empirical evidence that leaves many people skeptical on the role of religion in assisting people to recover from substance dependency. When some evangelical programs report rates of success of 50% and higher, most experts in the field regard such claims as unscientific and a self-serving manipulation of data.[1] The end result is that religious proponents think that there is no need to prove that religion helps in drug and alcohol rehabilitation while secular people disregard the potential of religion in helping abusers improve their functioning and attaining abstinence. Some of the critics of faith-based substance abuse programs contend that the data purported by religious providers are not valid due to the following key factors: (1) religious programs selectively accept (cream off the top, e.g., regression to the mean) clients, accepting only those who show good prospect of success, (2) outcomes are not assessed for clients who drop out of treatment, or those who do not maintain contact with the program following discharge, (3) finally, religious programs often define success in a non-standardized fashion using religious terminology, and rarely collect valid collateral data such as urinalysis results.

With the exception of AA groups (Fowler, 1993; McCrady & Miller, 1993), public service providers are not attempting to introduce religiously-based interventions or religiously-based components into an already existing public drug and alcohol service. It is important to note that AA can be offered on a continuum from having an evangelical emphasis to having an emphasis on non-sectarian social support–a fact that is rarely studied. To this end, none of the studies that have used spirituality interventions has contributed sufficiently to persuade society at large that spirituality and religion should be a value-added component of substance abuse interventions. Although programs that use spiritual approaches may be extremely helpful for clients, these programs are not available for every person in the community attempting to abstain from substances. Inclusion of a valid religiously-based module or program as one option of a public drug and alcohol program could be a significant opportunity to expand the number and type of treatment services available in the wider society.

Using RCCT to Study Faith-Based Substance Abuse Rehabilitation

To be able to assess the relationship between faith-based intervention and substance abuse rehabilitation we ought to establish and evaluate the effectiveness of spirituality and religion in a community-based, publicly funded drug and alcohol treatment setting using a RCCT. The use of RCCTs in the field of substance abuse has been promoted to examine the effectiveness of medications such as methadone and clonidine in the treatment of heroin and cocaine (Kahn, Mumford, Rogers, & Beckford, 1997; Lin, Strang, Su, Tsai, & Hu, 1997; Pozzi, Conte, & De Risio, 2000). Other studies apply RCCT to a theoretical counseling-based intervention (see for example, Liddle et al., 2001; Sandahl, Herlitz, Ahlin, & Röönnberg, 1998; Shakeshaft, Bowman, Burrows, Doran, & Sanson-

Fisher, 2002). The novelty in the approach proposed in this paper is to apply this rigorous method of effectiveness evaluation to a social transformational approach rather than biobehavioral interventions and more so to use it to compare the effectiveness of two compatible social interventions, one using religiously-based components and one not.

A RCCT could be proposed to compare two modes of case management for substance abusers: (1) traditional case management (comparison), and (2) religious-intensive case management (experiment). The hypothesis studied is that clients who receive intensive case management that links clients with spiritual and religious resources will, on average, demonstrate improved levels of functioning and reduced substance abuse as compared with clients in the comparison group who will receive standard intensive case management.

If the results show that spiritual/religious-intensive case management provides better outcome results, it will open the door for the selective incorporation of spirituality and religion as a legitimate mode of service and possible funding for drug and alcohol public programs throughout the United States. If, however, the results show that spiritual/religious-intensive case management provides lesser outcome results, it will be a cautionary note to service providers regarding the real efficacy of faith-based intervention in the public sector. The results of such study may help decide whether or not to integrate faith-based interventions into other areas of social service practice. Moreover, it could open the door for religious and spiritual based services to partner with existing public health services in a manner that provides clients with increased opportunities for access to various types of care.

The interaction between public and religious services can be viewed on a two-by-two matrix. On the one side is the provider and on the other side, the content of service. Thus, a provider can serve both secular and or religious components of service to clients who are or are not religious. In reality, however, secular providers (mostly public or publicly-funded services) provide mostly or only secular services regardless of clients' preferences). Consequently, no one study of secular providers has attempted to introduce a component of religious services into the regular public drug and alcohol services. As Miller et al. (1997) noted: "it is not clear how changes in spirituality and changes in substance abuse are related." These authors concluded that based on our knowledge, "the role of spirituality should be examined in relation to initial experimentation with alcohol and other drugs, establishment of regular use, development of problems and dependence, and recovery. Longitudinal study designs would be important in investigating such relationships over time" (p. 75).

Muffler, Langrod, and Larson (1992) recommended that clearly, not all substance abusers can be reached, much less successfully treated, by way of religiously oriented programs. This approach merits serious consideration; however, for individuals with a high degree of religious motivation, it has produced positive results comparable to those of other accepted forms of treatment (p. 584). In other words, a special faith-based program is appropriate for some people, but not all. What can apply to all is adding an available religious component to regular publicly funded substance abuse programs if it is found effective. In other words, if all clients receive the same mode of drug and alcohol intervention and only a randomly selected group receive an additional dosage of religious care than the impact of the dosage of religion services can be assessed as an addition to an existing social intervention.

What follows is a conceptual proposal on how to randomly assign individuals who volunteer for drug and alcohol services in a public health system regardless of the individual's spiritual/religious experiences and beliefs. For illustrative purposes, it is assumed that Phase 1 and Phase 2 clinical trials have already been performed and the results of these trials indicated that clients who received the proposed intervention found the intervention to be helpful and there were positive behavioral changes potentially associated with the proposed intervention.

Implementation of a Phase 3 Randomized Controlled Clinical Trial Setting

The setting for the proposed two-year study involves the use of federal and state block grant funding implemented in a county system responsible for the administration of public funds to become the point of care for all local residents who seek treatment services for drug and alcohol abuse and dependence. With decreased federal and state support, there will be many local and state governments willing to participate in such a study to lower the cost of caring for people who abuse substances. No matter which local government is selected to undertake this clinical trial, local substance abuse treatment service providers in this county will be used to provide outpatient drug and alcohol counseling services to assure a natural setting and to assure that upon completion of the RCCT the client continues to have available local drug and alcohol rehabilitation services. The setting described above is commonly utilized in our national public health service system to deliver drug and alcohol services to public sector clients.

Case Management

It is proposed that all clients who receive outpatient counseling services would be assigned to a case manager to assist them in the recovery process. In this study, case management services will be the intervention component that is manipulated as either standard case management or spiritual based case management.

Case management (CM) services have been increasingly incorporated in the delivery of substance abuse treatment services. Although there are no national standards on who is eligible for CM services, the model of CM services, the length of CM services, etc., these services are often utilized for individuals to help them obtain services to assist in their recovery of substance abuse and utilize community services effectively. In the context of drug and alcohol rehabilitation, a case manager may help the client engage in a number of different types of service activities and help the client get motivated to undergo a major behavioral change. Examples include linking the client to an AA group, motivating clients to engage in work activities, encouraging family members to support the person in rehabilitation, and assisting in securing financial and social benefits such as public housing (Cnaan, 1994). Case managers are usually people with a college degree who undergo a few weeks of on-the-job training for their position. It is common for each case manager to have a caseload of 10 to 25 clients depending on the intensity of care. Usually, eight case managers are supervised by one qualified social worker.

Proposed Intervention

The proposed study is a two-group design, pre/post test intervention in which both groups receive standard outpatient drug and alcohol counseling. Standard services are defined as once a week; one-on-one counseling and group counseling sessions will be available to all clients. All clients will also receive case management. Clients randomized to the comparison condition will receive standard treatment and intensive case management. Clients randomized to the experimental condition will receive the standard counseling services, and intensive case management with the option of a spiritual/religious context.

All clients will be enrolled in out-patient drug and alcohol treatment services. Each client will receive case management services for up to a six-month period. At the conclusion, case management and counseling services will be terminated. In Pennsylvania, the majority of patients assigned to outpatient counseling are engaged in counseling services for six months or less.

Intervention Conditions

All clients will receive standard drug and alcohol treatment services delivered by local licensed outpatient drug and alcohol treatment facilities. The amount, frequency, and duration of drug and alcohol counseling sessions will vary based on client need and will not be modified for the purpose of this study. The licensed treatment facilities will provide individual and group counseling services as well as an optional 12-step group (such as AA or NA). In an effort to control for the number of drug and alcohol treatment sessions provided, we will review client records and ask clients to report the total units of drug and alcohol treatment delivered by the treatment program. At a minimum, clients will receive one (1-hour) individual counseling session per week and one (1 and 1/2 hour) group counseling session. At a maximum, clients will receive one (1-hour) individual counseling session per week and 12 hours of group counseling.

The two groups studied will have in addition to these existing base services: (1) *Standard Case Management Sessions (Standard)*: In the comparison group, clients will also be assigned a drug and alcohol case manager who will provide standard case management services from a strength-based perspective. Clients in this condition will be eligible to receive case management services for up to 26 weeks, consisting of at least an hour of case management contact each week. To control for the type, frequency, and quantity of Standard Case Management services provided, the case manager will be required to deliver services using a structured interview (Zanis, 2006), the Needs and Progress Assessment Profile (NPAP) which helps guide the course of case management delivery. Importantly, the content of case management will review the following basic areas of client functioning: medical, employment, substance abuse, family, psychiatric, legal, and other needs (i.e., financial, housing, food, and goal planning). (2) *Spiritual/Religious Case Management Sessions (experimental condition)*: In the experiment group, clients will be provided with the exact same frequency of services, quantity of services and type of services outlined in the Standard condition. However, it will differ in one specific aspect. The structured NPAP interview will contain an additional area of client functioning titled "spirituality." When clients identify that they have a need to receive assistance in helping them to better understand their level of spirituality, the case manager will provide spiritual services. The R.E.S.T. model will be the experimental approach to providing spiritual services and only the case managers assigned to this mode of intervention will be trained to use it.[2] In addition to the spiritually-based interaction with the case manager, each client will get an offer to be linked with local-church faith mentors trained to counsel people with addictions.

The clients assigned to the experimental condition will also receive a minimum dose of three spirituality units (delivered through a standard intervention manual) in an attempt to adequately assess spiritual needs, understand client resources, and educate participants about the possible benefits of engaging in a spiritually-based treatment protocol as specific to their personal beliefs. The duration of a single unit is designed to be approximately 60 minutes in length. The duration of the spirituality intervention will be up to 26 weeks. If a client is interested in participating in additional spiritually-based services, the case managers will facilitate weekly individual or group meetings for clients to share religious experiences and to explore their spirituality as a tool in enhancing recovery. If the client is not interested in including spirituality as a dimension in his/her recovery, no further spirituality services will be provided by the case manager beyond the initial 3 sessions. Yet, the client will remain in the experimental condition and no crossover between groups will be allowed. Similarly, clients in the standard case management condition will not be allowed into the experimental group or be permitted to receive spiritual/religious services as facilitated by the case manager. Please note, these clients would be permitted to seek these services on their own.

In addition to religious discussions, the religious component will consist of caseworkers whose function is to help the client integrate spirituality in his/her recovery and to be linked with a religious supporting community. This will involve a number of tasks (doses of service) including: (1) assessment of baseline level and type of spirituality through individual meetings, (2) integration of community-based spirituality resources (linking clients with a locally-trained faith mentor), (3) spirituality motivation, (4) discussion of spirituality in one-on-one counseling, and (5) case consultation with the treatment provider agency to coordinate treatment efforts. These services will be provided at varying doses.

One approach is to assess the success group of clients in the treatment plus religion services (experimental group) as compared with the other group who receives only regular treatment (comparison group). Alternatively, the types of services and amount of religious care provided can be studied as a means to assess how much is enough of religious care. Importantly, since there does not exist evidence as to what an appropriate dose of spirituality is to effect change, clients will have an opportunity to receive varying hours of professional spirituality services each week. Additionally, clients will be encouraged to integrate community spirituality services in their treatment. In addition clients will be encouraged to use community-based (including congregations) supportive services. This information will be documented. The caseworker will record the length and type of service provided, as well as the general content of the service.

The client may choose to discontinue participating in spiritually-based services at any time, similar to their decision to discontinue participation in employment, or housing, or medical services. If the client chooses to continue in spiritually-based services, the role of the case managers will be to link clients with religious groups, congregations, and others in the community who share similar spiritual beliefs. Moreover, it will be the responsibility of the spiritual case manager to network within the community and identify spiritually-based support services to assist clients in the experimental condition.

The following inclusion/exclusion criteria have been established: (1) must be between ages 18 and 65, (2) must live in the selected county, (3) must have a DSM-IV substance abuse/dependence diagnosis and have used a substance within the past 30 days prior to admission, (4) must voluntarily consent to participate in the research project and to be randomized to one of the three treatment conditions (experimental group, comparison group or no treatment), and (5) must be appropriate to participate in an out-patient setting for drug and alcohol treatment services.

Exclusion criteria: The following exclusion criteria have been established for an individual which: (1) although 18 years of age, is enrolled in high school, (2) is presently receiving case management through another county-based social service agency, (3) is unable to commit to remain in the area during the next year, or (4) is having active, non-substance induced hallucinations.

Assessments: Subjects in both treatment conditions would complete the same data collection protocols including pre-treatment assessments, during treatment assessments, and post treatment assessments. For the proposed project, our post treatment assessment would be a simple 6 month follow-up interview that assesses various levels of client functioning such as substance use, mental health, employment, and spirituality. Broad dimensions of client change are included in the assessment to enable the research team to capture possible benefits of the experimental condition.

Similarly, qualitative interviews with subjects in the experimental condition would be conducted at the end of the project. These interviews would focus on the value of the experimental condition with the client, case manager and treatment staff. Specific attention would focus on how and if the intervention helped to achieve the outcomes. Exploration on the adequacy of the dose and duration of intervention services would be undertaken. The purpose of these qualitative interviews is to obtain verification about the program with an understanding of the clients' perspective on cause and effect. These interviews would also help shape the development of the intervention should a stage 3 trial be warranted.

PROJECT OUTCOMES

In addition to success in abstinence at defined time periods post enrollment into treatment, a number of secondary hypotheses will be generated for the project. Expected analyses include an understanding of the extent and nature of service utilization patterns. For example, how many clients reported a need for spiritual/religious services? What proportion of clients engaged in spiritual/religious services? How were these services provided? Did clients find these services helpful in assisting them to make changes? Was the spirituality of clients affected by these services? What types of changes were facilitated by spiritual/religious services? How did the case managers deliver services? What did the case managers report as important causal issues in helping to facilitate change? Was there a dose/response effect associated with condition? Within condition was there a dose/response effect in terms of service utilization? Was the case manager able to develop effective community based partnerships with spiritual/religious communities? Clearly, the proposed study can serve multiple uses.

If the above outcomes suggest a cause and effect relationship, then a proposed stage 4 randomized controlled clinical trial involving several communities would be warranted. Prior to the stage 4 trial, appropriate changes would be made to the intervention condition to implement changes and modifications in the intervention approach. Issues such as protocol development would be reviewed and modified. A stage 4 trial would have a significantly larger, more diverse sample from which subjects are recruited to participate. Hypotheses would be formulated prior to the study implementation and appropriate statistical calculations would be performed to determine optimal study size.

CONCLUSIONS

In an era in which politicians, policy makers, and the public at large are debating the role religiously-based social services can serve in society, there is a need for critical evaluation and documentation of the impact of religiously-based social services. The question is whether the spirit of religion coupled with public support can yield better results than comparable secular services.

How can we arrive at reliable studies on the impact of religious services after years of academic neglect? The key operative word for providing empirical proof is: *ceteris paribus*. In other words, a study ought to be carried out using the most rigorous tools modern science has to offer and one that controls for most threats to internal and external validity. For this purpose, it is recommended that social-science applications of the most rigorous and robust mode of study available in the biomedical and social service intervention filed namely randomized controlled clinical trials (RCCT). This method of research is presented along with the many threats to reliability and generalizability it aims to minimize or even eliminate. Understanding the many factors that can interfere in the assessment of spiritual and religiously-based social intervention highlights the need for applying RCCT in careful impact assessment.

This chapter concludes with a concrete proposal detailing how RCCT can be applied in studying a religiously-based social service intervention. The example shows that such an endeavor is possible and that within three to four years of study, a preliminary but definite answer to the question about the impact of religion in social service intervention can be obtained. RCCTs are complex and expensive, but the implications are significant in advancing the state of knowledge that this field deserves.

While the described stage 3 trial does not address all possible rival hypotheses regarding cause and effect relationships, it does advance our knowledge. However, caution is warranted in fully accepting the results of the above study. There are a number of methodological limitations to the project that merit discussion. Assuming that the faith-based experimental group would yield better results than the comparison group, one alternative explanation is that those in this group were offered more options and hence tailored a better program for themselves. In other words, it is not the faith-based intervention, but the many options that contributed to the outcome. Two caveats should be introduced in such a case. First, a careful researcher may replicate the stage 3 trial or design a stage 4 study based on the results obtained from the one proposed here, but in which the secular group is offered many more options. Such RCCT will provide us with information on whether it is the faith-factor or the option-factor that contributed to success. Second, and more importantly, regardless of the cause of greater effectiveness, including the faith-based option could be a more cost-effective and tax-payer friendly under the assumed outcome of greater services effectiveness.

Given the current movements in public funding shifts, it is time for the government and large foundations to step in and support the application of RCCTs in faith-based social services provision. The example in this article focused on substance abuse rehabilitation, but RCCT can be used in most social service fields. The more evaluative studies, the better and more refined will be our knowledge as to the efficacy of faith-based programs.

NOTES

1. Teen Challenge is an excellent example of a promising practice that was evaluated a few times without meeting most of the criteria of field study listed above. According its Website, Teen Challenge provides 3,400 beds for residential treatment in the U.S., and is privately funded. It is a faith-based, self-accrediting ministry with 98 accreditation standards its affiliates must fulfill. Its staff members have training in theology, rather than social work or medicine, because its approach is that of a ministry. Teen Challenge claimed a 70-86% cure rate for addiction. This rate is based on a few studies that did not apply any random selection or comparison group design. The most commonly mentioned studies are by Hess in 1975 and a doctoral dissertation in 1999 by Bicknese. Furthermore, these studies did not account for the many Teen Challenge members who did not complete the program and who are not invited to Teen Challenge's last step in Central Pennsylvania. Finally, Teen Challenge cannot be compared to any other program, as its clients are not offered any alternative care. What about not receiving anything? If only 25% are allowed to the last step and of them about 80% are "rehabilitated," then the real rate of success is only 20%.

2. R.E.S.T. (Rational Emotive Spiritual Therapy) is a case management-counseling modality that combines cognitive counseling with eight faith-based interventions such as meditation and scripture reading. Its three basic tenants are that (1) unwanted

behavior is changed by changing the beliefs and thoughts that support the unwanted behavior; (2) in order to sustain new wanted behaviors, new beliefs and thoughts must be identified and adopted; and (3) spiritual (faith-based) thoughts best replace the beliefs and thoughts that supported the unwanted behavior. R.E.S.T. was developed by Dr. Rick McKinney and applied with ex-prisoners in the Philadelphia area. For more information see; http://www.restcounseling.com/

REFERENCES

Allison, P. (1995). *Survival analysis using the SAS system: A practical guide.* Cary, NC: The SAS Institute Inc.

Barrett, M. E., Simpson, D. D., & Lehman, W. E. K. (1988). Behavioral changes of adolescents in drug abuse intervention programs. *Journal of Clinical Psychology, 44,* 461-473.

Bicknese, A. T. (1999). *The teen challenge drug treatment program in comparative perspective.* Unpublished doctoral dissertation. Northwestern University, Political Science Department. Evanston, IL.

Boruch, R. F. (1997). *Randomized experiments for planning and evaluation: A practical guide.* Thousand Oaks, CA: Sage.

Bracht, G. H., & Glass, G. V. (1968). The external validity of experiments. *American Educational Research Journal, 5,* 437-474.

Bradley, C. (1997). Psychological issues in clinical trial design. *Irish Journal of Psychology, 18* (1), 67-87.

Brinberg, D., & McGrath, J. E. (1985). Validity and the research process. Beverly Hills, CA: Sage.

Brody, B. A. (1998). *The ethics of biomedical research.* New York: Oxford University Press.

Campbell, D. T. (1969). Reforms as experiments. *American Psychologist, 24,* 409-429.

Campbell, D. T., & Rouso, M. J. (1999). *Social Experimentation.* Thousand Oaks, CA: Sage.

Campbell, D. T., & Stanley, J. C. (1963). *Experimental and quasi-experimental designs for research.* Chicago: Rand-McNealy.

Cnaan, R. A. (1994). The new American social work gospel: Case management of the seriously mentally-ill. *British Journal of Social Work, 24,* 533-557.

Cnaan, R. A., Boddie, S. C., & Wineburg, R. J. (1999). *The newer deal: Social work and religion in partnership.* New York: Columbia University Press.

Cook, T., & Campbell, D. T. (1979). *Quasi-experimentation.* Boston: Houghton-Mifflin.

Donahue, M. J. (1985). Intrinsic and extrinsic religiousness: Review and meta-analysis. *Journal of Personality and Social Psychology, 48,* 400-419.

Fowler, J. W. (1993). Alcoholics Anonymous and faith development. In B. S. McCrady & W. R. Miller (Eds), *Research on Alcoholics Anonymous: Opportunities and Alternatives* (pp. 113-135). New Brunswick, NJ: Rutgers Center of Alcohol Studies.

Gorsuch, R. L. (1995). Religious aspects of substance abuse and recovery. *Journal of Social Issues, 51,* 65-83.

Greenhouse, J. B., Stangl, D., & Bromberg, J. (1989). An introduction to survival analysis: Statistical methods for analysis of clinical data. *Journal of Counseling and Clinical Psychology, 57*, 536-544.

Hess, C. B. (1975). *Teen Challenge training center: Research summation.* Also a report for the National Institute on Drug Abuse (1976). *An evaluation of the Teen Challenge treatment program.* Washington, DC: United States Department of Health, Education and Welfare.

Johnson, B, R. (2002). *Objective hope, assessing the effectiveness of faith-based organizations: A review of the literature.* Philadelphia, PA: University of Pennsylvania, Center for Research on Religion and Urban Civil Society.

Kahn, A., Mumford, J. P., Rogers, G. A., & Beckford, H. (1997). Double-blind study of lofexidine and clonidine in the detoxification of opiate addicts in hospital. *Drug and Alcohol Dependence 44*, 57-61.

Kazdin, A. E. (1992). *Research design in clinical psychology.* Needham Heights, MA: Allyn & Bacon.

Koenig, H.G., McCullough, M.E., & Larson, D.B. Handbook of Religion and Health. New York: Oxford University Press, 2001: 18.

Liddle, H. A., Dakof, G.A., Parker, K., Diamond, G. S., Barrett, K., & Tejeda, M. (2001). Multidimensional family therapy for adolescent drug abuse: Results of a randomized clinical trial. *The American Journal of Drug and Alcohol Abuse, 27*, 651-688.

Lin, S., Strang, J., Su, L., Tsai, C., & Hu, W. (1997). Double-blind randomised controlled trial of lofexidine versus clonidine in the treatment of heroin withdrawal. *Drug and Alcohol Dependence, 48*, 127-133.

McCrady, B. S., & Miller, W. R. (1993). *Research on Alcoholics Anonymous: Opportunities and alternatives.* New Brunswick, NJ: Rutgers Center for Alcohol Studies.

Meinert, C. L., & Tonascia, S. (1986). *Clinical trials: Design, conduct and analysis.* New York: Oxford University Press.

Miller, W. R. (1990). Spirituality: The silent dimension in addiction research. *Drug and Alcohol Review, 9*, 259-266.

Miller, W. R. (1997). Spiritual aspects of addictions treatment and research. *Mind/ Body Medicine, 2*, 37-43.

Miller, W. R. et al. (1997). Addictions: Alcohol/drug problems. In: D. B. Larson, J. P. Sawyers, & M. E. McCullough. (Eds.), *Scientific research on spirituality and health: A consensus report* (pp. 68-82). Rockville, MD: National Institute for Healthcare Research.

Muffler, J., Langrod, J. G., & Larson, D. (1992). "There is a balm in Gilead": Religion and substance abuse treatment. In J. H. Lowinson, P. Ruiz, R. B. Milliman, and J. G. Langrod (Eds.), *Substance Abuse: A Comprehensive Textbook* (pp. 584-595). Baltimore: Williams & Wilkins.

Orr, L. L. (1999). *Social experiments.* Thousand Oaks, CA: Sage.

Pozzi, G., Conte, G., & De Risio, S. (2000). Combined use of trazodone-naltrexone versus clonidine-naltrexone in rapid withdrawal from methadone treatment. A comparative inpatient study. *Drug and Alcohol Dependence 59*, 287-294.

Rossi, P. H., Freeman, H. E., & Lipsey, M. W. (1999). *Evaluation: A systematic approach (5 Ed.).* Newbury Park, CA: Sage.

Sandahl, K., Herlitz, G., Ahlin, G., & Röönnberg, S. (1998). Time-limited group psychotherapy for moderately alcohol dependent patients: A randomized controlled clinical trial. *Psychotherapy Research, 8,* 361-378.

Shakeshaft, A. P., Bowman, J. A., Burrows, S., Doran, C. M., & Sanson-Fisher, R. W. (2002). Community-based alcohol counseling: A randomized clinical trial. *Addiction, 97,* 1449-63.

Teen Challenge. Official homepage. Downloaded from the Internet on August 22, 2003, from: http://www.teenchallenge.com/main/information/index.cfm?doc_id= 147

Zanis, D. General Issues Prior to Study Implementation. In Alexander, L., B., & Solomon, P. (Eds.) *The Research Process in Human Services: Behind the Scenes* (pp. 20-40). Canada. Thomson Brooks/Cole.

Zanis, D. (2006). The Needs and Progress Assessment Profile: A Method for Assessing the Needs of Substance Abuse Clients. Presented at the Society for Social Work Research Conference, San Antonio, TX. January 14, 2006.

Chapter 6

Testing Faith:
Improving the Evidence Base
on Faith-Based Human Services

Robert L. Fischer
Judson D. Stelter

SUMMARY. The U.S. federal government, through Charitable Choice, has opened public funding for the delivery of social services to faith-based organizations (FBOs) more than ever before. This increased access to governmental funding at all levels has led to a closer examination of the evidence base on the effectiveness of the services provided

Robert L. Fischer, PhD, is Research Associate Professor at the Center on Urban Poverty & Social Change, Mandel School of Applied Social Sciences, Case Western Reserve University. He specializes in the use of evaluation methods in applied human service settings. Judson D. Stelter, MSSA, is Research Assistant at the Center on Urban Poverty & Social Change, Mandel School of Applied Social Sciences, Case Western Reserve University.

Address correspondence to: Robert L. Fischer, Mandel School of Applied Social Sciences, Case Western Reserve University, 10900 Euclid Avenue, Cleveland, OH 44106-7164 (E-mail: fischer@case.edu).

This paper was originally prepared for the conference on Evaluation Methods & Practices Appropriate for Faith-Based and Other Providers of Social Service. Bloomington, IN: Indiana University, October 3-4, 2003.

[Haworth co-indexing entry note]: "Testing Faith: Improving the Evidence Base on Faith-Based Human Services." Fischer, Robert L., and Judson D. Stelter. Co-published simultaneously in *Journal of Religion & Spirituality in Social Work* (The Haworth Pastoral Press, an imprint of The Haworth Press, Inc.) Vol. 25, No. 3/4, 2006, pp. 105-122; and: *Faith-Based Social Services: Measures, Assessments, and Effectiveness* (ed: Stephanie C. Boddie, and Ram A. Cnaan) The Haworth Pastoral Press, an imprint of The Haworth Press, Inc., 2006, pp. 105-122.

by FBOs, and the capacity of FBOs to respond to data needs for accountability and program improvement efforts. This paper discusses the current status of evaluation research on FBO services and the emerging data needs among faith-based providers. Promising avenues for enhancing the current understanding of outcomes of FBO services are explored such as (1) adopting outcome measurement practices in use within the current nonprofit sector, and (2) developing more rigorous research designs tailored to the special contexts of faith-based services. The paper suggests an agenda in which FBO operators, funders, and evaluators work together to move forward in improving the evidence base on faith-based services.

KEYWORDS. Faith-based organizations, social services, evaluation methods, outcome monitoring

The Bush Administration's Faith-Based and Community Initiative seeks to give faith-based organizations (FBOs) equal footing with secular organizations in securing federal funding for the delivery of social services. One mechanism for furthering this goal, the Compassion Capital Fund (CCF), involves $105 million allocated between 2002-2004 to support capacity building, research, and evaluation of FBO practices. The CCF recognizes that FBOs are "uniquely situated" in serving "families in poverty, prisoners reentering the community and their families, children of prisoners, homeless families, and at-risk youth" (U.S. DHHS, 2002). It is in these programmatic areas that distinct increases in funding availability for FBOs have occurred. Beyond the CCF, much more federal funding is being awarded to FBOs through routine funding programs operated by an array of federal departments. For example, in FY 2004, approximately $2 billion in competitive grants across seven federal agencies were awarded to faith-based organizations, accounting for over 10 percent of the total funding awarded (White House, 2005).

The expanded role for FBOs within the domain of federally-funded human services carries with it increased scrutiny about the capacity and operational effectiveness of these organizations. It has even been suggested that FBOs, because of their religious characteristics, are being subjected to more scrutiny than their secular counterparts that receive federal funds (Manhattan Institute, 2002). Regardless of the motivations behind any special attention that FBOs receive, these organizations need to move forward with an agenda of establishing systems for the purposes of accountability, program improvement, and demonstrating effectiveness.

STATUS OF RESEARCH ON FAITH-BASED SERVICES

Overall, due to the relative youth of the FBO research field, there is a paucity of systematic data on FBO services and their effectiveness. Much of the research work on FBO services that is available is largely descriptive in nature, with a focus on programmatic models, delivery styles, and funding streams of FBO services (Independent Sector, 2003). Given this, there is a substantial and immediate need for increased emphasis on the evaluation and monitoring of the outcomes of FBO services. Currently, there are a number of important studies underway or that are beginning to report early findings. These studies reflect a commitment to the systematic study of FBO services and their effectiveness and recognition of the special circumstances surrounding the conduct of field research with these providers and their clients.

The Administration for Children and Families, through the Compassion Capital Fund, funded five studies that commenced in late 2002 and early 2003, results from which are pending. In addition to the CCF-funded studies, there are several notable projects that have recently released research reports on their work. First, a major study of the implementation of the Charitable Choice provisions of PRWORA over three years in three states has added much to the existing knowledge base (Kennedy & Bielefeld, 2003). The study component assessing the relative effectiveness of providers shows that, based on regression models applied to observational data, faith-based and secular providers achieve similar rates of job placement and wage rates among the clients they serve (Deb & Jones, 2003). The authors also report that FBO clients acquired jobs with fewer hours of work and less health insurance coverage, in part because FBOs may have had weaker referral networks.

A second study of note is an evaluation of Amachi, a model mentoring program for children of prisoners in Philadelphia based on a partnership between secular and faith-based organizations (Jucovy, 2003). The Amachi program adopted the outcome model used by Big Brother Big Sisters (BBBS), which previously demonstrated that positive results for mentees begin to occur after 12 months of engagement. Using this benchmark, 62 percent of Amachi matches were active 12 months or longer and reported higher retention compared to the BBBS program (62% vs. 46%).

A third study released recently is Monsma and Soper's (2003) comparative evaluation of welfare-to-work programs in Los Angeles. The authors selected 17 programs and then collected participant-level data from the selected programs. Based on this analysis, participants in the for-profit programs generally had fewer barriers while those in faith-based/integrated programs generally had more barriers. In terms of outcomes, the study found that faith-based/integrated programs were the least successful in placing unemployed participants into jobs by 6 and 12 months, but somewhat more effective in helping employed participants retain their employment.

Another useful study involves the InnerChange Freedom Initiative (IFI), a faith-based pre-release program for prisoners operated in Richmond, Texas (Johnson & Larson, 2003). The program includes in-prison bible-based programming and 6-12 months of aftercare while the participant is on parole. The authors implemented a matched group design, whereby outcomes for IFI participants could be contrasted with three comparison groups of prisoners who approximated the IFI group in important ways. Overall, the study found that IFI participants showed equivalent or slightly more recidivism than the three comparison groups on measures of re-arrest and incarceration within two years of release (p.17).

The studies of FBO services that are now emerging or underway represent the vanguard of work in the field and hold great promise for advancing the evidence base on faith-based human services. As yet, there are insufficient empirical studies from which to gauge a pattern of results. Moreover, the study and assessment of FBO services can be complex and should be conducted with recognition of the existing practical and analytical pitfalls.

CHALLENGES TO THE EVALUATION OF FBO SERVICES

Several challenges to evaluating the effectiveness of FBO services stem from the fact that many FBOs are small nonprofits and have limited capacity for ongoing data collection or systematic research studies (Fischer, 2004). In addition, due to the role of faith in these programs and how faith may impact service delivery, outreach, and outcomes, there is an added overlay of challenges to such field research. Two specific issues that may require attention are: (1) the role of selection bias in this context, and (2) dealing with analytic challenges.

Any evaluation study of faith-based services should consider the role of selection bias in the outcomes observed. This selection bias is largely manifest in two ways. First, research on "organic" religion demonstrates that religious participation and belief are related to a wide range of positive social and health outcomes (Johnson, 2002; Johnson & Siegel, 2003; Johnson, Tompkins, & Webb, 2002; Powell, Shahabi, & Thoresen, 2003; Wilcox, 2002). For example, youth with more religious involvement show better academic progress (Regnerus, 2002), and are more likely to engage in a range of healthy behaviors (Wallace, 2002). Given this, and postulating that within any given target population (e.g., ex-prisoners, drug addicts) individuals who seek out faith-based services may possess greater belief or openness to a faith alternative, then there may exist a self-selection bias among clients who volunteer for services delivered by FBOs (Kramer, Finegold, De Vita, & Wherry, 2005). For example, Heslin, Andersen, and Gelberg (2003) found that homeless women with no religious affiliation were half as likely to use faith-based services as women with a Christian affiliation. Such a selection bias among the population of individuals who seek, choose, or otherwise accept services from a faith-based service provider could have multiple and potentially contradictory effects on the program outcomes.

Another issue of concern in evaluating FBOs relates to the analytic tactics used to assess program success in the faith-based arena. One example is the analysis of subgroups of individuals that may exhibit selection biases beyond the initial selection bias reflected in their choice to participate in a faith-based program. Individuals who complete a FBO program are more likely to show greater success than non-completers on a range of outcome measures related to the program intent. For example, in the InnerChange Freedom Initiative (IFI) study, program graduates demonstrated dramatically lower recidivism rates over two years compared to non-completers [17% vs. 50% on re-arrest and 8% vs. 36% on incarceration, respectively] (Johnson & Larson, 2003). Such evidence, however, should be tempered by the realization that the experiences of completers does not generalize to all participants in faith-based services. In fact, if we adopt an intent-to-treat approach to the analysis, then the overall assessment of program efficacy must include the data on all participants, regardless of their level of program engagement. Despite this concern, the contrast between completers and non-completers may be important from a programmatic stance. Examining the characteristics of those who complete and do not complete may suggest whom the program engages most successfully. For example, in the case of IFI, program graduation was more frequent among Hispanic men, men over 35 years of age, and men judged to be at low risk, compared to the other categories of participants (p. 18).

It should also be noted that caution should be exercised in the analysis and presentation of findings as it is easy for some audiences to misinterpret reported findings. In a *Wall Street Journal* editorial, under the heading "Jesus Saves," the overwhelmingly positive results for IFI *completers only* were reported and followed with "(a)ll this, no doubt, will be profoundly discomforting to those who like the results but don't like religion" (*Wall Street Journal*, 2003). This was problematic in that it appeared that some were interpreting data from IFI completers as representative of the all participants. This and other reporting led to subsequent criticism that the results were being purposely misinterpreted (Kleiman, 2003). In the political context of the federal funding of FBOs, it would be beneficial to ensure the clarity of analyses and reporting of findings, both in the research domain and the popular press.

THE CURRENT NEED FOR DATA
ON THE FAITH-BASED SECTOR

The ongoing debate over the President's Faith-Based and Community Initiative involves a range of concerns but continues to include a heavy emphasis on the effectiveness of FBO services compared both to their secular counterparts and/or to no service at all (DiIulio, 2002). The Independent Sector's Measures Project surveyed over 900 nonprofit and religious organizations about a range of agency practices, including record-keeping and measuring outcomes (Wiener et al., 2002). The study found that a majority of nonprofits and religious congregations do regularly collect information and report on the effects of some of their programs, but this is usually in terms of outputs not outcomes. The Working Group on Human Needs (2003) issued a report supporting "... the conduct of independent, relevant, rigorous, and non-partisan research that compares outcomes of a wide range of approaches, including faith-based, secular, and other national and community-based organizations and programs" (p. 35).

Though there is a strong emphasis on working to increase the capacity of FBOs through promoting internal development and external support via intermediary organizations, more attention to these issues is needed. The most promising avenues for responding to the data needs regarding FBOs are through improving and expanding FBO data collection practices and fielding more rigorous comparative studies to address issues of effectiveness.

ADAPTING OUTCOME MONITORING METHODS FROM THE SECULAR NONPROFIT SECTOR

One opportunity for growth in the faith-based sector comes in the form of borrowing from the experience of secular nonprofits in engaging in outcome measurement activities. Though rigorous demonstrations are needed to determine the relative effectiveness of FBO services, other alternatives offer a viable avenue to aid FBOs in improving their programs and monitoring their success. One such alternative is the use of secular outcome measurement techniques, such as those that have been infusing the nonprofit sector in the U.S. since the mid-1990s, particularly among United Way-funded programs. The advent of outcomes measurement has spurred a major shift in the way nonprofits view themselves and the way they communicate their role to their funders, clients, and other stakeholders (Fischer, 2001). The Compassion Capital Fund National Resource Center (2005) has recognized the value of this approach and has produced a manual on outcomes measurement for use by intermediary organizations in their work with FBOs. The manual covers such topics as creating a program logic model, developing performance indicators and data collection methods, and creating a sustainable system for outcome measurement. The broader experience base that exists can offer valuable assistance to FBOs in at least two areas: (1) clarifying program theory and goals, and (2) specifying essential data and collection methods.

Clarifying Program Theory and Goals

There have been a variety of typologies put forward for characterizing faith-based and community-based programs (e.g., Monsma & Mounts, 2002; Sider & Unruh, 2004; Smith & Sosin, 2001; Working Group on Human Needs, 2002). Working Group (2003) defines an FBO as "any entity that is self-identified as motivated by or founded on religious conviction" (p. 2). The difficulty is generally not in distinguishing between faith-based and nonsectarian programs, but rather in distinguishing among faith-based services in respect to role of faith. Scott, Montiel, Keyes-Williams, and Han (2003) summarize the existing typologies and identify two forms–(1) size and geographical typologies, and (2) level of institutionalized faith typologies. Institutionalized faith typologies attempt to assess the relative presence of faith in the program based on attributes such as organizational structure, administrative factors, environmental/physical characteristics, funding sources, and program activities/services (Scott et al., 2003).

The ability to assess the relative degree of faith intensity of a social service program is central to clarifying the program's theory, logic, and key outcomes (Hatry, Van Houten, Plantz, & Greenway, 1996). A core tactic in this work is the development of an elementary program logic model that specifies the basic elements of the program and its intended outcomes. Such schematic program depictions can aid program operators in maintaining a unifying focus and ensuring that all necessary data elements are being collected.

Much like the ability to measure the "dose" of services received (e.g., in terms of length, frequency, and extent of participation), measuring faith intensity allows for examination of the comparative effect of more or less faith in a program area. The operators of faith-based programs likely have a clear expectation about the role of faith in their program theory and, ultimately, in participant success. Loconte and Fantuzzo (2002) interviewed operators of 37 FBOs that target at-risk youth and found that ". . . they consider exposure to religious values and beliefs a crucial part of their strategy for helping needy kids–and structure their programs accordingly" (p. 10). Given the frequent belief that faith can be "a" or "the" key ingredient in some type of programs, it is essential to explicitly address this dimension in evaluation efforts.

A critical factor here is to assess the presence of faith in the program, as it is experienced by the program participants, recognizing that the level of religious content in a program can be very different from the religious nature of the host organization. The Working Group on Human Needs (2003) developed a typology with five categories for faith-based programs: faith-permeated, faith-centered, faith affiliated, faith-background, and faith-secular partnerships. By design, the typology identifies ". . . the visibly expressive ways that religion may be present in a community-serving organization or program. Classifications are based primarily on observable and explicit manifestations of religion, such as language, symbols, policies, and activities (p. 29). For instance, 'explicitly religious' program content is identified by 'activities and verbal messages that are, on their surface, intrinsically religious (such as prayer, study of sacred texts, discussions of religious doctrine, worship services, invitations to personal religious commitments, etc.)' " (p. 29).

For example, elements of interest would include a religious program name, use of religious facilities or accoutrements, use of religious language, concepts, or explicitly religious activities within the program itself. The assessment would not include the religious sponsorship or funding of a program if participants would not be routinely aware of these factors. However, Ebaugh, Pipes, Chafetz, and Daniels (2003) report that in a sample of FBOs, 84 percent used some type of religious imagery in the "public face" of the organization, such as through organizational names, logos, and mission statements (p. 416). This suggests that in a large proportion of FBOs, the faith attributes as experienced by program participants should be associated with the image the program presents to the public. In terms of practical usefulness of such faith indices, Bielefeld, Littlepage, and Thelin (2003) demonstrate that a quantitative scale of faith influence can be used to create meaningful subgroups of programs under study. In their study of TANF-funded employment services in Indiana, the authors developed an eight-point scale of faith influence and then created three program categories: not influenced by faith (zero points), moderate faith influence (1-4 points), and strong faith influence (5-8 points). Bielefeld et al. (2003) used the program groupings to identify interesting contrasts between the types based on various factors related to organizational functioning and service delivery.

Specifying Essential Data and Collection Methods

The broader nonprofit sector, along with pertinent nonprofit literature, can aid FBOs in identifying what participant-level data are needed and how best to collect it. A recent example of this comes in the evaluation of the Amachi program, where faith-based providers collaborated with Big Brothers Big Sisters, and adopted the well-regarded evaluation tools and methods developed by BBBS in the assessment of Amachi's mentoring operations and outcomes (Jucovy, 2003).

The data needs for FBOs may extend beyond the kinds of participant service information that many nonprofits have grown accustomed to reporting (e.g., client background characteristics, counts of participants and services delivered). The types of data needed by FBOs require thinking through the program management and decision making processes that may lie ahead. For example, FBOs likely will want to monitor the characteristics of the individuals who seek out, or enroll in, their services to gauge the need for program changes. The data needed to inform this process will include basic demographic and socio-economic data, but may also require baseline assessments of the client's condition or need. Similarly, program operators often need to monitor the amount of services delivered in a given period (e.g., monthly), and may wish to have these service statistics broken out according to program location or staff member. Aggregate service statistics, however, are not useful in understanding the service experience of any one client or subgroups of clients. For this process, client-level data can be summarized to show program managers how the overall program experience of participants may be shifting.

Beyond the identification of data elements, another challenge facing FBOs where they can benefit from the experience of secular programs is in the area of data collection. The practical difficulties of securing data from participants can be a formidable obstacle for many small agencies and programs. A useful practice for any program attempting to set up an ongoing data collection system is to investigate the practices of similar programs. Much of the difficulty arises in how to embed the data collection activities into the normal functioning of the program without leading to a disruption of the participant's experience of the program. For FBOs approaching the task it is useful to examine the key contact points where data collection can or should occur. In most human service programs there are four points at which data are generally collected: (1) Baseline: data are collected at the participant's first contact with or intake to the program and baseline data are essential for tracking clients and their progress; (2) In-program: data are kept on the services received by the participant and their flow through the program and can be useful for assessing service delivery; (3) Exit: data are collected upon the client's graduation, termination, or last contact with the program. Exit data are useful for tracking pre to post changes but can be problematic when programs experience high drop-out rates; and (4) Follow-up: data are collected some time after the participant's exit from the program to assess the participant's view of the services and/or any further changes in the participant's status or condition. Follow-up data are very useful but can be difficult for many programs to collect due to resource limitations and/or problems in locating participants after contact has ended. The tailoring of data collection approaches to individual programs will require a full examination of the program model and its scope, the target population, and the resources available for data collection activities. In all these areas, FBOs can learn from the experiences of secular nonprofits that have spent time developing workable data collection approaches.

IMPLEMENTING MORE RIGOROUS EVALUATION DESIGNS

In the evaluation of any human service intervention, it is widely accepted that the use of randomized research designs (well-implemented) lead to the most credible assessments of program impact. Experimental and quasi-experimental research designs have the distinct advantage of eliminating the role of a range of plausible intervening factors that could rival the program itself in explaining observed impacts (Cook & Campbell, 1979). See article by Zanis and Cnaan in this volume for additional discussion of randomized designs in this context. The use of random assignment in conducting an experimental study of faith-based services involves multiple ethical and operational challenges. Two principal issues arise related to the role of randomization in human service programs. First, in instances where individuals are to be randomized either to a treatment or control condition (Tx vs. C), an ethical issue arises in that some individuals are denied the service in order to create an equivalent no-service control group. Second, in instances where individuals are to be randomized to alternative treatments (T1 vs. T2), the issue involves the assignment of individuals with a strong treatment preference to a condition they do not desire. In the case of FBOs, the idea that, for example, a "faith-averse" person would be randomly assigned to a faith-intensive program is not only impractical but also likely to result in higher attrition rates among individuals whose did not receive their preferred assignment. Corrigan and Salzer (2003) addressed the conflict between random assignment and treatment preference and discussed the impact of treatment preference on study recruitment, engagement in the intervention, and attrition. To combat these problems they proposed a design wherein only those individuals with no treatment preference are randomized to conditions. Volunteers with a strong treatment preference are simply assigned to that desired service option.

One option is to assess the relative effectiveness of program variations so that no no-service control group exists and thereby no volunteers are denied service. Rather, the design now uses random assignment to sort volunteers into two or more program variations. For example, prisoners who volunteer for faith-based services might be randomly assigned to three program options that vary in regard to intensity (e.g., high, moderate, or mild faith emphasis). A principal limitation of this design is the absence of a "no-cause" baseline; that is, without a true control group, there are no data on the gross effect of any of the interventions (Cook & Campbell, 1979). Also, consequently, larger samples are needed to detect the presumably smaller outcome differences between the alternative treatments.

Other designs have been proposed in the literature but examples of their use have not been widely reported. For example, Moberg, Piper, Wu, and Serlin (1993) proposed a two-step nested randomized assignment wherein there is selection between two treatment options with the understanding that they may still be randomly assigned to the control group. Further, Braver and Smith (1996) proposed their "combined modified" design for voluntary treatments. After recruitment, subjects are randomized to be *invited* to participate in one condition only (e.g., T1, T2, or C). Within each group (e.g., those assigned to be invited to T1), some subjects will agree to participate and others will refuse. An additional group is composed of those invited to participate in a lottery among the various conditions. Those agreeing to the lottery are then randomly assigned to the various study conditions. If successfully implemented, the combined modified design offers many interesting group comparisons while still minimizing the ethical issues associated with an experimental design.

One avenue for implementing a more rigorous design would be to use a mixed design that involves both random (R) and nonrandom (NR) elements. (See Figure 1.) In this example, assignment of individuals is done according to some baseline assessment of their level of openness to and preference for faith-based services. Openness to faith-based services is likely related to religious background and current participation, personal belief, etc. By sorting clients according to treatment preference the design avoids the problems of cross-assignment as discussed earlier. In the example, individuals are systematically sorted into three groups: (1) faith-disposed = prefer FBO service/unwilling to accept secular service, (2) faith-indifferent = no marked preference between FBO and secular service, and (3) faith-averse = prefer secular service/unwilling to accept FBO service.

Once sorted according to their stated disposition, participants could be assigned to research groups through random assignment. Faith-disposed individuals could be randomized into two faith-based program alternatives (e.g., more vs. less intensive). Faith-averse individuals could be randomized into two secular alternatives (e.g., individual vs. group model). Faith-indifferent individuals could be randomized into either a faith-based or a secular alternative; this would allow for the most direct comparison of faith-based and secular services within a relatively homogenous group of target participants. Further, each of the three arms of the design could be expanded to include a no-service control group, if

FIGURE 1. Schematic of Proposed Design Incorporating Both Treatment Preference and Randomization Elements.

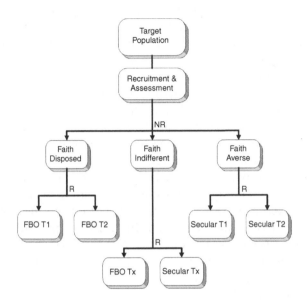

the ethical issues associated with this approach have been adequately addressed.

A benefit of the design is that it includes several useful elements: relative effectiveness studies of programs offered to individuals with relatively strong faith preferences and a comparative study of faith-based versus secular programs for individuals with no preference. In addition, it capitalizes on the full recruitment sample by assigning all volunteers to some part of the study.

While this model, if implemented, may provide invaluable data for the evaluation of FBOs, it is not without its limitations. At a very practical level, it is unclear how evenly participants might be dispersed by faith preference as they self select. With a topic so personal and emotion-laden as faith or the volitional absence thereof, it is uncertain how many participants would identify as being indifferent to a faith-based service. Preliminary evidence from a study of TANF recipients involved with job training services in an urban center found a somewhat even distribution. Among 149 TANF recipients involved in an interview study, 30 percent reported a preference for a faith-based program,

21 percent reported a preference for a non-faith-based program, and nearly one-half (48%) reported no preference. Additional empirical work on this issue would be helpful, especially an examination of how the distribution may be impacted by the outreach strategies and intake points used by programs. In addition, there may well be an interaction effect between faith preference and program type that would need to be considered. For example, if faith-averse individuals happen to prefer individual-focused programs, this will result in that program option appearing to be distinctly more effective than a group-based option.

Another concern relates the accuracy of the design's portrayal of the process by which participants engage services of different types. At the community level, the ability of participants to have a true choice among a range of service providers may be constrained by the local market for services and the contracting relationships of government entities. While Charitable Choice provisions require that participants be notified of their right to access an alternative non-FBO service provider, a recent study by Kramer, Finegold, De Vita, and Wherry (2005) has raised concerns about how this provision is implemented at the local level. As such, more attention to the choice process is needed before this design could be used effectively.

Another final issue is the extent to which faith-based programs seek to cause individual participants to engage in a more religious, faith-centered lifestyle. Such "faith outcomes" can be central to the underlying theory and belief of FBO services, but may exist as outcomes that are outside of the program's public logic model. For example, a program may seek to help former cash welfare recipients secure employment through job search counseling and assistance in completing a GED. Regardless of whether the program is faith-based or secular, the operators will collect data on participants' completion of the GED and success of job search activities. However, GED completion and job search activities might not be the only dimensions a FBO is concerned with in regards to effectiveness. In the faith-based program, the program model may call for increasing participants' religious behaviors and spiritual openness as an important end in itself, but also as a mechanism to propel individuals to success on the educational and employment outcomes. Given that religious participation is found to be associated with a range of decreased risks and enhanced protective factors that accrue to the individual (Hester, 2002), it is challenging to tease apart the programmatic aspects that may influence the identified outcomes.

FUTURE DIRECTIONS

The notion of funding FBOs with federal dollars to provide social services has been met with both support and skepticism, but to date many positions have not yet fully risen above conjecture. There is now a dramatic surge in the amount of attention and funding being directed to assessing the operation, impact, and effectiveness of faith-based services. Carrying out such evaluation activities requires capacity, resources, and supports that are currently not available to many small-scale FBOs. There is a specific need to increase FBOs' internal capacity to systematically collect data and use it for program monitoring and improvement activities. In this regard, FBOs might find their closest allies in their secular counterparts. A wide range of secular nonprofits have been working toward establishing data collection and analysis and could be a tremendous resource for FBOs in identifying approaches to adopt or adapt. One clearly successful example of moving in this direction comes in the form of the Philadelphia-based Amachi mentoring program where faith-based mentors collaborate with staff from Big Brothers-Big Sisters in monitoring the process and outcomes of mentoring. Simultaneously, the evaluation research community and funders of such efforts should expand the discussion of how to bring more resources (technical and financial) to bear on the evaluation needs of the faith-based sector. This effort should support and expand strategies to increase internal capacity for evaluation, as well as opportunities to engage in research with external partners that bring relevant expertise.

Though the experiences of secular nonprofits may be of great use to FBOs, faith-based providers are still faced with the unique need to define and quantify the role of faith in their programs. Bringing a level of clarity to characterization of *faith* in social service programs will lead to the empirical testing of the relative impact of faith. In addition, it is essential that future research incorporate more rigorous comparative designs in evaluating the efficacy of FBOs. Critical to the success of comparative designs are randomization methodologies which will be able to reduce and account for potential selection biases in FBO services. The expanded use of outcome monitoring practices by FBOs, along with the fielding of more rigorous comparative designs promise to lead to substantial enhancements in the evidence base on the operation and effectiveness of faith-based services.

REFERENCES

Bielefeld, W., Littlepage, L., & Thelin, R. (2003). Organizational analysis: The influence of faith on IMPACT service providers. In S. S. Kennedy and W. Bielefeld (Eds.), *Charitable choice: First results from three states* (pp. 65-86).

Braver, S. L., & Smith M. C. (1996). Maximizing both external and internal validity in longitudinal true experiments with voluntary treatments: The "combined modified" design. *Evaluation and Program Planning, 19*, 287-300.

Compassion Capital Fund National Resource Center. (2005). Measuring outcomes. Intermediary development series. Washington: U.S. Department of Health and Human Services. Available at http://www.acf.hhs.gov/programs/ccf/resources/gbk_pdf/om_gbk.pdf

Cook, T. D., & Campbell, D. T. (1979). In *Quasi-experimentation: Design and analysis issue for field settings*. Boston: Houghton Mifflin.

Corrigan, P. W., & Salzer, M. S. (2003). The conflict between random assignment and treatment preference: Implications for internal validity. *Evaluation and Program Planning, 26*, 109-121.

Deb, P., & Jones, D. (2003). Does faith work? A preliminary comparison of labor market outcomes of job training programs. In S. S. Kennedy and W. Bielefeld (Eds.), *Charitable choice: First results from three states* (pp. 57-64).

DiIulio, J. (2002, Fall). The three faith factors. *The Public Interest*, 50-64.

Ebaugh, H. R., Pipes, P. F., Chafetz, J. S., & Daniels, M. (2003). Where's the religion? Distinguishing faith-based from secular social service agencies. *Journal for the Scientific Study of Religion, 42*, 411-426.

Fischer, R. L. (2004). The devil is in the details: Implementing outcome measurement in faith-based organizations. *Nonprofit Management & Leadership, 15*(1), 25-40.

Fischer, R. L. (2001). The sea change in nonprofit human services: A critical assessment of outcomes measurement. *Families in Society, 82*, 561-568.

Hatry, H., Van Houten, T., Plantz, M., & Greenway, M. (1996). *Measuring program outcomes: A practical approach*. Alexandria, VA: United Way of America.

Heslin, K. C., Andersen, R. M., & Gelberg, L. (2003). Use of faith-based social service providers in a representative sample of urban homeless women. *Journal of Urban Health, 80*, 371-382.

Hester, R. D. (2002). Spirituality and faith-based organizations: Their role in substance abuse treatment. *Administration and Policy in Mental Health, 30*, 173-178.

Independent Sector. (2003). *The role of faith-based organizations in the social welfare system–A report on the 2003 spring research forum*. Retrieved September 3, 2003, from http://www.independentsector.org/PDFs/srf03report.pdf

Johnson, B. R. (2002). *A better kind of high: How religious commitment reduces drug use among poor urban teens*. Philadelphia: University of Pennsylvania, Center for Research on Religion and Urban Civil Society.

Johnson, B. R. (2004). Religious programs and recidivism among former inmates in prison fellowship programs: A long-term follow-up study. *Justice Quarterly, 21*(2), 329-354.

Johnson, B. R., & Larson, D. B. (2003). *The InnerChange Freedom Initiative–A preliminary evaluation of a faith-based prison program.* Philadelphia: University of Pennsylvania, Center for Research on Religion and Urban Civil Society.

Johnson, B. R., & Siegel, M. B. (2003). *The great escape–How religion alters the delinquent behavior of high-risk adolescents.* Philadelphia: University of Pennsylvania, Center for Research on Religion and Urban Civil Society.

Johnson, B. R., Tompkins, R. B., & Webb, D. (2002). *Objective hope–Assessing the effectiveness of faith-based organizations: A review of the literature.* Philadelphia: University of Pennsylvania, Center for Research on Religion and Urban Civil Society.

Jucovy, L. (2003). *Amachi: Mentoring children of prisoners in Philadelphia.* Philadelphia: Public/Private Ventures and the University of Pennsylvania Center, for Research on Religion and Urban Civil Society.

Kennedy, S. S., & Bielefeld, W. (Eds.). (2003). *Charitable choice: First results from three states.* Indianapolis: Indiana University-Purdue University Indianapolis, School of Public and Environmental Affairs, Center for Urban Policy and the Environment.

Kleiman, M. A. R. (2003, August 5). Faith-based fudging: How a Bush promoted Christian prison program fakes success by massaging the data. *Slate.* Retrieved on September 10, 2003 from http://slate.msn.com/id/2086617/

Kramer, F. D., Finegold, K., De Vita, C. J., & Wherry, L. (2005). *Federal Policy on the Ground: Faith-Based Organizations Delivering Local Services.* Discussion Paper 05-01. Washington: The Urban Institute. July.

Loconte, J., & Fantuzzo, L. (2002). *Churches, charity, and children–How religious organizations are reaching America's at-risk kids.* Philadelphia: University of Pennsylvania, Center for Research on Religion and Urban Civil Society.

Manhattan Institute. (2002, May 21). *The Jeremiah project.* Address given at the 2002 Second Annual Lecture on the State of Religion and Public Life. Retrieved on September 4, 2003 from http://www.manhattan-institute.org/html/sor2002.htm

Moberg, D. P., Piper, D. L., Wu, J., & Serlin, R.C. (1993). When total randomization is not possible: Nested random assignment. *Evaluation Review, 17,* 271-291.

Monsma, S. V., & Mounts, C. M. (2002). *Working faith: How religious organizations provide welfare-to-work services.* Philadelphia: University of Pennsylvania, Center for Research on Religion and Urban Civil Society.

Monsma, S. V., & Soper, J. C. (2003). *What works: Comparing the effectiveness of welfare-to-work programs in Los Angeles.* Philadelphia: University of Pennsylvania, Center for Research on Religion and Urban Civil Society.

Powell., L. H., Shahabi, L., & Thoresen, C. E. (2003). Religion and spirituality: Linkages to physical health. *American Psychologist, 58*(1), 36-52.

Regenerus, M. D. (2002). *Making the grade–The influence of religion upon the academic performance of youth in disadvantaged communities.* Philadelphia: University of Pennsylvania, Center for Research on Religion and Urban Civil Society.

Scott, J. D., Montiel, L. M., Keyes-Williams, J., & Han, J. S. (2003, June). *The scope and scale of faith-based social services: A review of the research literature focusing on the activities of faith-based organizations in the delivery of social services (2nd ed.).* Albany, NY: SUNY-Albany Rockefeller Institute of Government, The Roundtable on Religion and Social Welfare Policy.

Sider, R. J., & Unruh, H. R. (2004). Typology of religious characteristics of social service and educational organizations and programs. *Nonprofit and Voluntary Sector Quarterly, 33*(1), 109-134.

Smith, S. R., & Sosin, M. R. (2001). The varieties of faith-related agencies. *Public Administration Review, 61,* 651-670.

U.S. Department of Health and Human Services. (2003). *CCF funded research.* Retrieved September 4, 2003 from http://www.acf.hhs.gov/programs/ccf/citizens/citz_resrch/citz_resrch.html

U.S. Department of Health and Human Services. (2002, June). *The Compassion Capital Fund and the Faith- and Community-based Initiative, HHS fact sheet.* Retrieved on September 4, 2003 from http://www.hhs.gov/news/press/2002pres/20020605.html

Wallace, J. M. (2002). *Is religion good for adolescent health? A national study of American high school seniors.* Philadelphia: University of Pennsylvania, Center for Research on Religion and Urban Civil Society.

Wall Street Journal. (2003, June 20). Jesus saves: How President Bush found himself hugging a murderer in the White House. Editorial. Retrieved September 10, 2003 from http://www.opinionjournal.com/taste/?id=110003652

White House. (2005, March 1). Grants to Faith-Based Organizations FY 2004. Washington: Office of Faith-Based and Community Initiatives. Retrieved June 9, 2004 from http://www.whitehouse.gov/government/fbci/final-report.pdf

Wiener, S. J., Kirsch, A. D., McCormack, M. T., Weber, M. A., Zappardino, P. H., & Collyer, C. E. (2002). *Balancing the scales: Measuring the roles and contributions of nonprofit organizations and religious congregations.* Washington, DC: Independent Sector.

Wilcox, W. B. (2002). *Good dads–Religion, civic engagement, & paternal involvement in low-income communities.* Philadelphia: University of Pennsylvania, Center for Research on Religion and Urban Civil Society.

Working Group on Human Needs and Faith-Based and Community Initiatives. (2003). *Harnessing civic and faith-based power to fight poverty.* Washington, DC: author.

Working Group on Human Needs and Faith-Based and Community Initiatives. (2002). *Finding common ground: 29 recommendations of the working group on human needs and faith-based and community initiatives.* Washington, DC: author.

Zanis, D. A., & Cnaan, R. A. (2006). Social service research and religion: Thoughts about how to measure intervention-based impact. *Journal of Religion & Spirituality in Social Work.*

SECTION II

EMERGING EMPIRICAL FINDINGS

Introduction

Stephanie C. Boddie

Ram A. Cnaan

The conceptual section, as a whole, suggests that we need very rigorous and quite expensive studies to be able to answer the most pressing public policy dilemmas of the early 21st century: Are faith-based social services more effective than their secular counterparts? In the past decade since 1996, we have seen an increased reliance on faith-based social services and there is too little evaluation research to substantiate the claim that these two sectors are different in their organizational characteristics, and in their efficacy in helping people in need. We asked scholars who were engaged in studying this question to summarize their findings in a manner that would help us put some of the pieces together in the sector puzzle.

Our empirical studies section starts with a paper by Elizabeth A. Graddy (Chapter 7). One of the challenges when comparing faith-based social service providers with other providers is the issue of their organizational characteristics and organizational culture. While not much is known about these qualities, Graddy demonstrates, based on the directory of services in Los Angeles county, that faith-based providers are more specialized in certain service areas (food services, transitional services, recreation, and housing/shelter) than secular and public providers. Faith-based providers are more likely to provide counseling, yet not substance abuse or mental health counseling. Finally, they are more

[Haworth co-indexing entry note]: "Introduction." Boddie, Stephanie C., and Ram A. Cnaan. Co-published simultaneously in *Journal of Religion & Spirituality in Social Work* (The Haworth Pastoral Press, an imprint of The Haworth Press, Inc.) Vol. 25, No. 3/4, 2006, pp. 125-128; and: *Faith-Based Social Services: Measures, Assessments, and Effectiveness* (ed: Stephanie C. Boddie, and Ram A. Cnaan) The Haworth Pastoral Press, an imprint of The Haworth Press, Inc., 2006, pp. 125-128.

likely to be well distributed where poor and needy people reside. The challenge then is to control for these differences and make sure that assessment of effectiveness is sector-related and not characteristic-based.

Wolfgang Bielefeld (Chapter 8) uses data from a three-state evaluation of welfare to work programs. His first finding is that comparing programs in different states is tricky business as their regional cultures and local regulatory traditions differ dramatically, making cross-state conclusions questionable. In Indiana, job training providers and clients were interviewed. Like many evaluators, Bielefeld struggled with assessing the degree to which service providers were faith-based and the impact of this component on service outcome. Bielefeld used a pre- and post-service study to assess impact on clients. However, like others in this volume, he found that relying on service providers to administer the tests was too difficult and often impossible, thereby limiting the utility of the results. Finally, even this one-state study became difficult, as the state changed its funding priorities over the course of the study, thereby altering the provider system. Bielefeld shows that assessing efficacy can be done, but is quite complex and would be costly as it needs to be carried out solely by the researchers, in a relatively short period of time and at comparable sites.

Stephen V. Monsma (Chapter 9) is a veteran of faith-based social services evaluation. Monsma carried out the first ambitious study of four types of services in four cities with varying levels of religiosity in each organization. In this article, Monsma uses data from 17 Los Angeles welfare-to-work programs and their clients in order to assess the comparative effectiveness of faith-based and secular programs. The paper concludes that no single type of welfare-to-work program was more effective than another across the board. Instead, the different types of programs seemed to be particularly effective in certain specialized areas. The faith-based programs were especially effective in providing welfare recipients with emotional support and a sense of having a sympathetic, understanding support base. The for-profit providers were especially effective in providing needed training in marketable job skills and in helping to find employment. This article concludes that effectiveness can best be conceptualized in terms of program outcomes, and that such outcomes—while difficult to measure—can be measured with sufficient accuracy to justify the effort.

Jill Witmer Sinha (Chapter 10) approached the evaluation challenge from a different perspective. Sinha assessed the level of success of a church-based program for teenage drop-outs in North Philadelphia. Based on the success of an earlier project, six United Methodist churches were contracted to educate and care for teenagers who had dropped out. Like Bielefeld, Sinha found that relying on the congregations to collect data was problematic, and hence a large part of her planned data collection never materialized. While some of the studied congregations and their arrangements failed to deliver what they were contracted for, overall, the clients benefited from the service; they liked the providers and their services, and although services were provided in churches clients did not report any attempted proselytism.

Susan E. Grettenberger, John P. Bartkowski, and Steven R. Smith (Chapter 11) joined forces to study faith-based organizations in Washington, Michigan, and Mississippi. These authors conducted a series of comparative case studies regarding secular and faith-based providers in three different social service domains: (1) transitional housing, (2) parent education, and (3) residential substance abuse treatment programs. All case studies utilized the same research protocol.

David Campbell and Eric Glunt (Chapter 12) used examples from an evaluation of California's Community and Faith-Based Initiative (CFBI) to illustrate a research strategy that takes local networks as the primary unit of analysis. This approach focuses on understanding the roles various organizations play within local service delivery networks, and on analyzing how local actors coordinate services to affect participant, organization, and system outcomes. This undertaking aimed to overcome the drawbacks of comparing dissimilar organizations. They suggest that it may be more appropriate to begin thinking in terms of the concept of "network effectiveness," since the outcomes of value to participants and the public are the products of collaborations that involve many organizations. Like other researchers, they contend that the use of the network analysis is subject to a reliable definition of faith. Finally, they remind us that good evaluation research focuses simultaneously on process evaluation and outcome evaluation.

Finally, F. Ellen Netting, Mary Katherine O'Connor and Gaynor Yancey (Chapter 13) use grounded theory to analyze and report on a study based on 65 key informants in 15 promising faith-based organizations in four urban areas. They chatted with respondents to discover what made their direct service programs faith-based, and slowly a story emerged; the programs are motivated by mission-driven visions which are tied to forces beyond local programs and steeped in deep traditions. They found that while the expressed values of acts of faith are integral in the faith-based discussion, they do not tell the full story. The deep drivers of human behavior and practice are found in the specific beliefs and interpretations of individuals who are involved either as leaders or participants in faith-based organizations. This large-scale and intensive study that included researchers from four universities was selected to be the last one in this volume as it represents how little we know about faith-based organizations. It demonstrates what McGrew and Cnaan noted in the second chapter: when a field of study is neglected for such a long period of time it takes many years to really understand it and know what questions to ask and how to ask them.

Chapter 7

How Do They Fit?
Assessing the Role of Faith-Based
Organizations in Social Service Provision

Elizabeth A. Graddy

SUMMARY. Despite public policies that promote an increased role
for faith-based organizations in the delivery of publicly supported services, insufficient attention has been paid to assessing how service delivery by faith-based and secular providers might differ. This study
considers the issues involved in evaluating the role of faith-based organizations within the broad context of a community's social service offerings. Criteria are developed for assessing role differences by comparing
the types of services, delivery approaches, and service locations offered
by different types of providers. The approach is then illustrated using a
large sample of social service providers in Los Angeles County. Important
role differences are revealed. Faith-based organizations offer fewer and
different types of services than their secular counterparts. The results
suggest a modest and focused role for faith-based organizations in social service delivery, but one that is complementary to the efforts of

Elizabeth A. Graddy, PhD, is Professor and Director, Program in Public Policy,
School of Policy, Planning, and Development, University of Southern California, RGL
208, Los Angeles, CA 90089-0626 (E-mail: graddy@usc.edu).

[Haworth co-indexing entry note]: "How Do They Fit? Assessing the Role of Faith-Based Organizations
in Social Service Provision." Graddy, Elizabeth A. Co-published simultaneously in *Journal of Religion &
Spirituality in Social Work* (The Haworth Pastoral Press, an imprint of The Haworth Press, Inc.) Vol. 25, No.
3/4, 2006, pp. 129-150; and: *Faith-Based Social Services: Measures, Assessments, and Effectiveness* (ed:
Stephanie C. Boddie, and Ram A. Cnaan) The Haworth Pastoral Press, an imprint of The Haworth Press, Inc.,
2006, pp. 129-150.

secular providers. The methodological issues raised by such analyses are highlighted.

KEYWORDS. Faith-based organizations, public service delivery, social services, nonprofit organizations.

With the passage of the "Charitable Choice" provision of the 1996 Personal Responsibility and Work Opportunity Reconciliation Act, the institutional structure of social service delivery in the United States changed. The rules under which faith-based organizations (FBOs) may deliver publicly supported services changed to encourage an increased role for religious organizations in social service delivery. If states contract with nonprofit organizations to deliver social services, they must now also include religious organizations as eligible contractees. The contracting religious organizations retain control over the expression of their religious beliefs (Center for Public Justice, 1997). The important public policy change is that organizations whose main activities are religious (e.g., congregations) may now receive money to support social services. Religiously affiliated organizations whose main purpose is the delivery of social services (e.g., Catholic Charities, Salvation Army) were not affected by this provision.

This policy change was expected to increase social service provision by congregations (Chaves, 1999; Cnaan and Boddie, 2001), but the Act seems to have signaled a broader change. There is evidence that states now *seek* to contract with FBOs. Several states, e.g., California (Anderson et al., 2000), Indiana (Kennedy and Bielefeld, 2002), and Texas (Yates, 1998), have encouraged FBOs to compete for public funding with other social service providers. The Act also prompted the interest of philanthropic foundations, and some began to direct funding accordingly (e.g., the Robert Wood Johnson's $100 million initiative to FBOs that operate volunteer programs to help elderly, disabled, or chronically ill individuals).

This promotion by public and private funders of an expanded role for faith-based organizations is taking place with little information on how service delivery by FBOs might differ from that of secular providers. What role can FBOs reasonably be expected to assume in the context of a community's social service offerings? Is this role consistent with the expected advantages of faith-based service delivery? Without a contextual understanding of the role of different types of service providers, it is unclear what contributions FBOs can or should be expected to make. I consider here the issues involved in such an assessment. What criteria should be used, and what are the associated methodological concerns?

In the next section, evaluative criteria are developed based on a review of expectations about faith-based service provision. Then, I illustrate this assessment approach and consider the associated methodological issues with an analysis of social service providers in Los Angeles County.

EVALUATION CRITERIA

Faith-based organizations have a long history of participating in social service delivery. Ram Cnaan (1999) observes that religious groups were virtually the sole providers of social services in the United States before the 20th century. This changed in 1935 with the Social Security Act, which began the transfer of responsibility for social services to the government. Social service delivery became more secular and professional. Nevertheless, religious groups continued to provide social services, although the nature and extent of their role is not well understood. With the advent of Charitable Choice and the Bush Administration's creation of an Office of Faith-Based and Community Initiatives, their role is expected to increase.

There may be good reasons to attempt to systematically increase the role of FBOs in social service delivery. The unique organizational structure of faith-based organizations may offer both efficiency and effectiveness advantages over secular service providers. First, FBOs may be more *efficient* at delivering some social services. Avenues for such an advantage include the role of churches and of volunteers. Churches are the most common institutions in many communities. As such, they have existing infrastructure and network relationships–buildings, human resources, community connections–that could be utilized for the delivery of social services. For example, Botchwey (2003), in a study of a small section of North Philadelphia plagued by urban blight, found that the majority of nonprofits operating in the neighborhood were congregations, and that the congregations had a longer history in the community than other types of nonprofits. Griener (2000) argues that congregations, because of such strong community connections, are well positioned to address the multi-service needs of the poor.

FBOs also have access to volunteers. This low-cost labor may enable FBOs to offer more services or to allot more time to each beneficiary than other service providers. The role of volunteers in the service provision of faith-based organizations is substantial. Printz (1998) found that D.C. congregations relied heavily on volunteers, with 230 congregations estimating that they used over 20,000 volunteers in 1996. Cnaan (1999) in his study of 113 congregations in six cities found that the monthly number of volunteer hours averaged 148 hours per program. These efficiency arguments suggest three evaluative criteria–the *number of locations*, with FBOs expected to provide more, the *number of services offered per location,* with FBOs expected to have a multi-service orientation, and *costs*, with FBOs expected to utilize volunteers to provide services at lower costs than secular providers.

Second, the defining characteristic of these organizations–their reliance on faith–may make them more *effective* either by leading them to employ different methods of service delivery, or to employ the same methods with more intensity than secular service providers. Several writers have noted that faith-based organizations typically see their work as a ministry or a calling, which causes them to behave differently than other service providers. Etindi (1999) identifies 3 differences. FBOs, because of their sense of mission, are more willing to make a long-term commitment to a service recipient, continuing to provide service until changes occur (see also Trulear, 2000). FBOs are more likely to rely on mentoring, one-on-one relationships in which a person is encouraged, challenged, and taught how to do things. Finally, faith-based organizations are more adaptive, more willing to conform services to an individual's needs, in contrast to a governmental program that requires all participants to conform to the program (see also Sherman, 2000). Bartkowski and Regis (1999) in their study of 30 Mississippi congregations found that those located in poor areas frequently adopted intensive and sustained interpersonal engagement as a primary service provision strategy. This effectiveness argument suggests *differences in service delivery methods* between FBO and secular providers as an evaluative criterion.

Finally, faith-based and secular providers may choose to provide different services. The discussion above suggests that FBOs may focus on services that require a long-term commitment and life-transforming effects. However, several studies (e.g., Printz, 1998; Cnaan, 1999; Grettenberger, 2000) have found that congregations most commonly provide short-term emergency services (food, clothing, and financial assistance). In addition, Chaves and Tsitsos (2001) in a study of

1236 congregations nationwide found that congregations do not tend to be involved in more than fleeting personal contact with needy people, nor did their services entail a particularly holistic approach to crosscutting needs, nor aim at character transformation. These findings suggest that the implications drawn from the faith-based mission may be incorrect. Rather than character transformation, congregations may view their role in service delivery as providing emergency services. Such services may offer the best fit for the expertise of their volunteers, and their available resources.

Alternatively, we may have an incomplete picture of faith-based service providers. The focus of these studies is limited to congregations. Thus, the picture they suggest of the service provision patterns of the broader population of service-providing FBOs may be misleading. It may be that congregations choose to focus on a narrower set of services than FBOs in general since service provision is not their primary purpose. Therefore, differences in *services provided*–both among types of faith-based providers and compared to secular providers–is an important criterion for understanding the potential contribution of different types of service providers.

To summarize, this discussion has identified 5 criteria for assessing the role of faith-based organizations in social service delivery–location, multi-service orientation, cost, delivery method, and types of service offered. To provide the most useful information, however, these criteria must be comparative. Analyses that consider only one provider type may identify patterns that represent the demand for services, rather than organizational differences in supply. This suggests the need for studies that place faith-based providers in a service delivery context. Such place-based analyses would allow comparisons of the delivery patterns of faith-based providers with their secular counterparts, while controlling for differences across communities in the needs for specific services and in preferences about their delivery.

The next section illustrates such an analysis with an exploration of a diverse set of social service providers in Los Angeles County. The methodological challenges raised in such assessments are highlighted.

ANALYSIS

This analysis considers the relative roles of faith-based and secular organizations in the delivery of social services by looking at a large sample of social service providers in Los Angeles County. The county, by any standard, is large and complex. It houses almost 10 million people, organized into about 90 incorporated cities and numerous additional neighborhoods, many of which are multiethnic. County residents have substantial social service needs, with large numbers who are poor, uninsured, and have limited education. Moreover, a substantial proportion of the population has only limited English-language skills. The size of the county and the extent of its needs guarantee the presence of social service providers in all economic sectors offering a large number of diverse services. These characteristics suggest that Los Angeles County offers a useful and interesting case from which to study organizational patterns in urban social service delivery.

The data upon which this study is based were provided by INFOLINE of Los Angeles County,[1] and represent a snapshot of active human service providers to Los Angeles County residents in 2000. INFOLINE's purpose is to provide referral services to those in need; thus, they make every effort to maintain a comprehensive and accurate database of human service providers.[2] They collect contact, location, and service offerings information on all public and nonprofit providers who have provided services for at least 6 months, are licensed as required, and have an independent governing body. For-profit providers are included only if their services are not adequately met by nonprofit or public organizations.

These data enable us to explore 4 of the 5 evaluative criteria identified in the previous section–multi-service orientation, location, types of services offered, and delivery method. The data do not include information on service costs. This assessment of the role differences of faith-based and secular service providers begins with an analysis of providers and the first two criteria. Then, service differences and the last two criteria are considered.

Providers

The sample of social service providers is large and diverse. Faith-based providers are self-defined as such, and the set includes organizations ranging from local congregations to large, national, religiously-affiliated organizations whose primary purpose is service delivery. Their secular counterparts are similarly diverse, ranging from small community-based organizations to large county agencies, and include public, secular nonprofit, and for-profit organizations.[3]

The data set contains 3461 service provider organizations offering 116 services. Providers can offer more than one service, and the resulting sample includes 5544 service delivery observations.[4] The distribution of providers by organizational type is summarized in Table 1, where FBO denotes faith-based organizations, SNP denotes secular nonprofits, PUB denotes public agencies, and FP denotes for-profit firms. The for-profit sector numbers should not be regarded as comprehensive, given INFOLINE's inclusion criteria, but are indicative of that sector's complementary role in service provision to vulnerable populations. In addition, note that these data do not allow us to assess the contributions of different types of providers *within* these broad organizational categories.[5]

These data provide a context for exploring the role of faith-based organizations in social service delivery. Among the 3461 service providers, 11% are faith-based, 47% are secular nonprofits, 35% are public, and 7% are for-profit. Thus, 82% of active social service providers in this Los Angeles County sample are either secular nonprofit or public.[6]

Multi-Service Orientation

Table 1 allows us to explore one of the hypothesized differences in service delivery by faith-based providers–an expected multi-service orientation. The table reveals that faith-based service providers offer more services on average (2.5) than their secular counterparts, which range from 1.1 by for-profit providers to 1.7 by secular nonprofit providers. Of the 5544 service offerings, FBOs provide 17%. Secular nonprofits provide 49%, public agencies provide 29%, and for-profit firms provide almost 5%. Thus, for this sample we find that FBOs do have a multi-service orientation. On average, they are less specialized than other organization types in their service offerings. This suggests that they have the ability to offer more integrated service delivery.

Location

A second hypothesized difference in service providers is in their locational choices. FBOs may locate in different neighborhoods than

TABLE 1. Service Providers by Organizational Type

	FBO	SNP	PUB	FP
Number of service provider organizations	388	1630	1216	227
Number of services offered	958	2727	1598	261
Average number of services offered per provider organization	2.5	1.7	1.3	1.1

other service providers making their services either more or less accessible to those who need them. It is difficult to assess whether there are in fact locational differences because of the large difference in the number of service locations by organizational type. For example, we expect to see secular nonprofit providers in the most areas as they have the largest number of service locations. Given that there are only 388 FBO locations in our data set, compared to 1630 for secular nonprofits, it cannot be that their coverage of the county is comparable. Some insight may be gained however, by viewing subsections of the county that differ in the prevalence of poverty.

The Los Angeles County Department of Health Services divides the County into 8 Service Planning Areas (SPAs) and provides demographic data on those areas (Los Angeles County Department of Health Services, 1999). The locations of service providers were mapped by zip code and organizational type. Consider here the two extremes. SPA 5 (West) is the least needy of the Los Angeles County SPAs. In 1997, only 7% of its population had income below the federal poverty line, only 5% were on welfare, and only 5% had less than a high-school level of education. SPA 6 (South) is, by these same indicators, the most needy. In 1997, 35% of its population had income below the federal poverty level, 16% were on welfare, and 40% had less than a high-school level of education. Figure 1 presents only nonprofit providers and denotes the location of SNP and FBO social service providers in these two areas. In SPA 5, secular nonprofit providers are located in almost every zip code, while FBOs are located in only a few zip codes in this relatively wealthy area. When one looks at the relatively poor SPA 6, however, the pattern is dramatically different. Both FBOs and secular nonprofits are present in every zip code in this area. This suggests that FBOs concentrate their limited resources in areas of greater need.

This mapping effort, however, is merely suggestive. Much more work is needed on locational choice before any conclusions can be drawn. In particular, the needs of the communities must be measured with considerably more precision. Wolpert, Seley, and Motta-Moss (2004)'s study of the locations of nonprofit organizations in New York City is an example of a more comprehensive analysis of the match between nonprofit facilities and neighborhood needs. They explore a variety of neighborhood characteristics including land use, population, ethnicity, income, and crime. Their analysis, while just focused on the nonprofit sector, revealed significant service gaps in lower income neighborhoods. Botchwey (2003) studied nonprofits operating in 7 contiguous census tracks in a poor area of North Philadelphia and found that faith-based

FIGURE 1

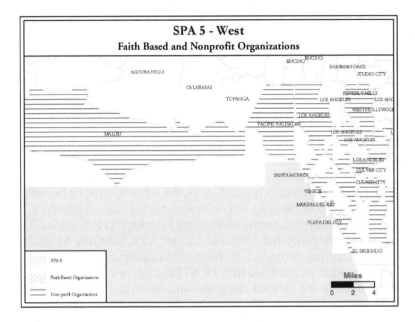

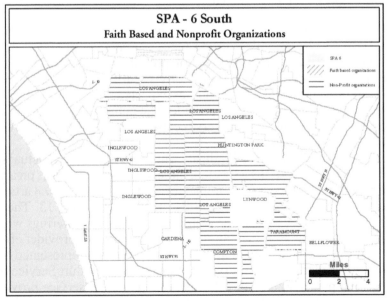

organizations were far more likely to be operating in the neighborhood than secular nonprofits. Moreover, congregations were distributed throughout the area, while secular nonprofits tended to be located close to major throughways. These studies reveal the usefulness of GIS mapping as a means to assess the coverage and responsiveness of different types of service providers.

SERVICES

The data set includes 116 different types of services, but many of these services are similar. To better understand whether different types of organizations focus on different kinds of services, a reclassification and aggregation scheme is needed. A useful scheme must be broadly accepted to allow comparisons in findings across studies. Therefore, I selected the National Taxonomy of Exempt Entities (NTEE) codes. These codes were created by the National Center for Charitable Statistics to categorize services provided by nonprofit organizations. The original 116 services were reclassified into 18 NTEE categories. The types of services included in the general categories are described in the Appendix.

Differences in Services Offered

This categorization allows us to examine differences between faith-based and secular providers in the types of services offered. Table 2 presents a crosstabulation analysis of providers by service category. The chi-square test reveals a statistically significant association (X^2 = 2341, significance level .000). Thus, as expected, service providers differ in the types of services they provide. The nature of that relationship is revealed by looking at actual versus expected counts, and the provider and service percentages.

The bolded cells in Table 2 indicate where the incidence of actual service provision exceeds the expected, indicating more emphasis on a service by a provider type. For example, the analysis predicted 9.8 arts and culture offerings by secular nonprofits; they actually had 13. The %-within-Provider row reveals the distribution of service offerings within each provider type, thus indicating the concentration of provider effort. For example, the provision of arts and culture services represented only .5% of all secular nonprofit services. Finally, the %-within-Service row reveals the percentage of all offerings of a particular service provided by each provider type. This is an indication of the relative role of each

TABLE 2. Provider*Service Crosstabulation

		Arts/ Culture	Business Services	Civil Rights	Community Improvement	Education	Environment/ Animals	Food	General Health	Housing/ Shelter
FBO	Count	**2**	**8**	**12**	**3**	38	1	**194**	50	**87**
	Expected	3.5	45.8	10.5	8.1	99.4	5.2	58.6	89.9	33.7
	% within PROVIDER	.2%	.8%	1.3%	.3%	4.0%	.1%	20.3%	5.2%	9.1%
	% within SERVICE	10.0%	3.0%	19.7%	6.4%	6.6%	3.3%	57.2%	9.6%	44.6%
SNP	Count	**13**	**148**	**37**	**34**	166	**16**	109	**332**	62
	Expected	9.8	130.3	30.0	23.1	282.8	14.8	166.7	255.8	95.9
	% within PROVIDER	.5%	5.4%	1.4%	1.2%	6.1%	.6%	4.0%	12.2%	2.3%
	% within SERVICE	65.0%	55.8%	60.7%	72.3%	28.9%	53.3%	32.2%	63.8%	31.8%
PUB	Count	5	15	11	10	**363**	**13**	36	104	45
	Expected	5.8	76.4	17.6	13.5	165.7	8.6	97.7	149.9	56.2
	% within PROVIDER	.3%	.9%	.7%	.6%	22.7%	.8%	2.3%	6.5%	2.8%
	% within SERVICE	25.0%	5.7%	18.0%	21.3%	63.1%	43.3%	10.6%	20.0%	23.1%
FP	Count	0	**94**	1	0	8	0	0	**34**	1
	Expected	.9	12.5	2.9	2.2	27.1	1.4	16.0	24.5	9.2
	% within PROVIDER	0	36.0%	.4%	0	3.1%	0	0	13.0%	.4%
	% within SERVICE	0	35.5%	1.6%	0	1.4%	0	0	6.5%	.5%
Total	Count	**20**	**265**	**61**	**47**	**575**	**30**	**339**	**520**	**195**
	% of Total	.4%	4.8%	1.1%	.8%	10.4%	.5%	6.1%	9.4%	3.5%

TABLE 2 (continued)

		Jobs	Mental Health	Other Human Services	Philanthropy Voluntarism	Public Protection	Public Safety	Social Benefit	Recreation	Youth Development	Total
FBO	Count	34	79	374	4	5	8	2	42	15	958
	Expected	62.0	119.2	256.1	12.6	49.8	15.6	30.6	38.2	19.4	
	% within PROVIDER	3.5%	8.2%	36.0%	.4%	.5%	.8%	.2%	4.4%	1.6%	100%
	% within SERVICE	9.5%	11.4%	25.2%	5.5%	1.7%	8.9%	1.1%	19.0%	13.4%	17.3%
SNP	Count	190	480	758	59	83	44	22	93	81	2727
	Expected	176.6	339.4	729.0	35.9	141.7	44.3	87.1	108.7	55.1	
	% within PROVIDER	7.0%	17.6%	27.8%	2.2%	3.0%	1.6%	.8%	3.4%	3.0%	100%
	% within SERVICE	52.9%	69.6%	51.1%	80.8%	28.8%	48.9%	12.4%	42.1%	72.3%	49.2%
PUB	Count	120	92	294	9	194	37	148	86	16	1598
	Expected	103.5	198.9	427.2	21.0	83.0	25.9	51.0	63.7	32.3	
	% within PROVIDER	7.5%	5.8%	18.4%	.6%	12.1%	2.3%	9.3%	5.4%	1.0%	100%
	% within SERVICE	33.4%	13.3%	19.8%	12.3%	67.4%	41.1%	83.6%	38.9%	14.3%	28.8%
FP	Count	15	39	56	1	6	1	5	0	0	261
	Expected	16.9	32.5	69.8	3.4	13.6	4.2	8.3	10.4	5.3	
	% within PROVIDER	5.7%	14.9%	21.5%	.4%	2.3%	.4%	1.9%	0	0	100%
	% within SERVICE	4.2%	5.7%	3.8%	1.4%	2.1%	1.1%	2.8%	0	0	4.7%
Total	Count	359	690	1482	73	288	90	177	221	112	5544
	% of Total	6.5%	12.4%	26.7%	1.3%	5.2%	1.6%	3.2%	4.0%	2.0%	100%

provider type within a service. For example, 65% of all arts and culture services are offered by secular nonprofits. So SNPs are the major providers of these services even though that provision represents a very small percentage of their overall service offerings.

Table 2 thus reveals service provision patterns for each of the provider types. *Secular nonprofit providers* offer the largest number of services, and have a larger than expected presence in 11 of the 18 service categories. This indicates a breadth of mission. They also strongly dominate offerings in a few of these services, e.g., philanthropy and voluntarism, community improvement, youth development and mental health, providing at least 70% of the service offerings.

In contrast, *faith-based organizations* have a higher than expected presence in only 5 types of services–food, housing/shelter, other human services, civil rights, and recreation. FBOs also do not dominate any service category to the extent that SNPs do, but they have a very strong role in food services, providing 57% of the service offerings. This represents 1 in 5 of all FBO service provisions. Other human services, however, represent their greatest focus, at 36% of all FBO service provisions.

Public organizations have a higher than expected presence in 7 types of services–social benefit, public protection, education, environment and animals, public safety, recreation, and job services. Many of these reflect the unique role of the public sector. As one would expect, they dominate in social benefit services, providing 84% of these service offerings. Education services, however, are the dominant focus within the sector. Twenty-three percent of all public sector offerings are of education services.

Finally, *for-profit firms* have a higher than expected presence in only 3 types of services–business services, health, and mental health services. They do not dominate in any service, but their greatest relative presence is in business services where they represent 36% of the offerings. These services are also their dominate interest representing 36% of all FP service offerings. For-profit organizations are the most limited in their breadth of service offerings. This presumably reflects the limitations in data collection noted earlier, as well as this sector's relatively limited presence in social services.

To summarize, we find clear differences in the types and ranges of services offered by different types of providers. The provision patterns of public agencies (around social benefit services) and for-profit firms (around business services) reflect the unique roles of those sectors. Within the nonprofit sector, faith-based organizations are far more concentrated in their service offerings than secular nonprofits. Faith-based organizations in Los Angeles County concentrate their presence in 5 types of services. Secular nonprofits have a strong presence in a much more comprehensive set of services.

Kearns, Park, and Yankowski (2005) also use NTEE codes to classify services in their study comparing faith-based and secular community service corporations in Pittsburgh. Although they do not use statistical significance tests in their paper, their data seem to suggest that Pittsburgh faith-based providers are more concentrated in other human services, housing, and food than are secular nonprofit providers. The use of similar taxonomies of services and appropriate statistical significance tests are necessary for comparisons across studies, and such comparisons will ultimately enable us to understand organizational and community differences in the role of different types of service providers.

Differences in Service Delivery Approaches

The taxonomy of social services enabled us to identify the general service foci of different types of provider organizations, but there may also be substantially different approaches to the delivery of services *within* these groupings. Two relevant hypotheses are suggested by the literature on faith-based service delivery. First, are FBOs more likely than other types of providers to provide transitional help? Second, are FBOs likely to use different methods than other types of service providers, thus building on their relative advantage as service providers? Consider each.

Transitional Assistance. As noted earlier, the empirical literature indicates that congregations, a major component of FBOs, focus their attention on transitional assistance. Here, this focus is considered within the broader context of social service providers. Services that are transitional in nature cross several of the general service categories analyzed earlier in this section. Eight services were identified: congregate meals, emergency food, and home-delivered meals from Food Services, shelter from Housing/Shelter Services, financial assistance, holiday assistance, and personal/household goods from Other Human Services, and disaster services from Public Safety. Of the 5,544 service provision observations, 815 (almost 15%) represent transitional assistance.

A provider*transitional service crosstabulation analysis is presented in Table 3. The chi-square test reveals a statistically significant relationship ($X^2 = 1457.2$, significance level .000) between provider type and whether or not transitional services are offered. As expected faith-based

TABLE 3. Provider*Transitional Services Crosstabulation

		Transitional Assistance	Other Services	Total
FBO	Count	**517**	441	*958*
	Expected	140.8	817.2	
	% within PROVIDER	54.0%	46.0%	*100%*
	% within SERVICE	63.4%	9.3%	*17.3%*
SNP	Count	245	**2482**	*2727*
	Expected	400.9	2326.1	
	% within PROVIDER	9.0%	91.0%	*100%*
	% within SERVICE	30.1%	52.5%	*49.2%*
PUB	Count	45	**1553**	*1598*
	Expected	234.9	1363.1	
	% within PROVIDER	2.8%	97.2%	*100%*
	% within SERVICE	5.5%	32.8%	*28.8%*
FP	Count	8	**253**	*261*
	Expected	38.4	222.6	
	% within PROVIDER	3.1%	96.9%	*100%*
	% within SERVICE	1.0%	5.3%	*4.7%*
Total	**Count**	815	4729	*5544*
	% of Total	14.7%	85.3%	*100%*

organizations are far more likely to offer these services than other providers. Note that they are the only provider type offering more transitional services than expected. FBOs offer 63% of all transitional assistance offerings even though FBOs provide only 17% of all social service offerings in our sample. Not surprisingly, these service offerings are also the major focus of the sector's efforts, representing 54% of the services offered by FBOs. This result is consistent with what previous studies have found. As noted earlier a focus on transitional services by FBOs may represent the best use of their unique resources. Volunteers can provide these services with little formal training. Moreover, neighborhood churches are well positioned locationally to identify and reach needy recipients.

Differences in service methods. The last comparison considered is the expectation that service providers will focus on different means of delivering services. Such an analysis requires that one disaggregate a service category and identify alternative methods. I do so here by examining mental health services. The relatively small role of FBOs in mental health services revealed in Table 2 is surprising given the expectation articulated in the literature that FBOs would have a comparative advantage in providing life-transforming services. It may be that organizations provide different types of services within the mental health services category that are in line with their relative strengths. Mental health services represent 690 observations in our data, and included 5 types of services–counseling and self help, mental health services and treatment, and substance abuse services and treatment. The provider*mental health services crosstabulation analysis is presented in Table 4. The chi-square test reveals a statistically significant relationship ($X^2 = 169.5$, significance level .000) between providers and the type of mental health services offered.

Table 4 reveals some interesting differences in mental health service provision. For-profit organizations focus on treatment offerings in both mental health and substance abuse, perhaps because these services are more likely than the others to be reimbursable by third-party insurers. Public providers focus on mental health services and treatment. It may be that the outcomes of these services are harder to measure than substance abuse services and thus the public sector may prefer to provide them internally rather than contract them out to private providers. Secular nonprofits conversely provide more substance abuse services and treatment. Finally, faith-based organizations provide more counseling and self-help programs and substance abuse treatment. This emphasis is quite consistent with the expected advantages of FBOs. Counseling and self-help efforts to solve mental health problems are services for which faith-based organizations have unique and appropriate expertise. In such services, volunteers can work one-on-one with service recipients and employ methods that draw directly on their religious orientation. This is in contrast to the trained professionals usually needed for mental health treatment.

This analysis thus reveals some of the expected differences in the service delivery foci of providers, as well as the complementary nature of these differences. Notably, in both of these analyses we see evidence that FBOs provide services that are not as likely to be funded by third-party insurers. Both public and private insurers provide funding to support drug and alcohol abuse and mental health treatment. Such support is less likely for counseling and self-help interventions. Similarly, transitional services are less likely to have consistent funding streams as compared to many of the other social services. The commitment by FBOs to providing transitional assistance may also include a commitment to

TABLE 4. Provider*Mental Health Services Crosstabulation

		Counseling/ Self Help	Mental Health Services	Mental Health Treatment	Substance Abuse Services	Substance Abuse Treatment	Total
FBO	Count	**47**	**5**	**3**	12	**16**	**83**
	Expected	23.5	17.9	4.8	26.2	10.6	
	% within PROVIDER	56.6%	6.0%	3.6%	14.5%	19.3%	100%
	% within SERVICE	24.1%	3.4%	7.5%	5.5%	18.2%	**12.0%**
SNP	Count	**136**	87	19	**172**	**62**	**476**
	Expected	134.5	102.8	27.6	150.4	60.7	
	% within PROVIDER	28.6%	18.3%	4.0%	36.1%	13.0%	100%
	% within SERVICE	69.7%	58.4%	47.5%	78.9%	70.5%	**69.0%**
PUB	Count	8	**51**	**6**	24	3	**92**
	Expected	26.0	19.9	5.3	29.1	11.7	
	% within PROVIDER	8.7%	55.4%	6.5%	26.1%	3.3%	100%
	% within SERVICE	4.1%	34.2%	15.0%	11.0%	3.4%	**13.3%**
FP	Count	4	6	**12**	10	**7**	**39**
	Expected	11.0	8.4	2.3	12.3	5.0	
	% within PROVIDER	10.3%	15.4%	30.8%	25.6%	17.9%	100%
	% within SERVICE	2.1%	4.0%	30.0%	4.6%	8.0%	**5.7%**
Total	Count	**195**	**149**	**40**	**218**	**88**	**690**
	% of Total	28.3%	21.6%	5.8%	31.6%	12.8%	100%

funding those services.[7] As such, the provision serves an important complementary role in social service delivery.

DISCUSSION AND CONCLUSION

I argue here that our efforts to understand the role of faith-based organizations in social service provision will be most productive if that role is analyzed within a specific service delivery context. Such place-based analyses make it easier to control for differences across communities in the needs for specific services and in preferences about their delivery. One can then compare the behavior of different types of service providers within the community to better understand their relative contributions.

This approach was illustrated with an analysis of Los Angeles County social service providers. Several methodological issues were raised in this analysis and other similar efforts to look at social service provision in the context of specific communities (e.g., Wolpert, Seley, and Motta-Moss, 2004; Kearns, Park, and Yankowski, 2005). We find that careful classification of types of services and of providers, a matching of demand or need characteristics of the community with the location of providers, and finally the use of appropriate statistical tools are needed if we are to increase our understanding of the roles of different types of service providers.

The Los Angeles study finds important differences in the service provision patterns of secular and faith-based organizations. Faith-based organizations offer more services per location than other types of providers, suggesting a multi-service orientation. But, FBOs are highly concentrated in their service offerings, which are primarily focused on the provision of food, housing/shelter, and other human services. This concentrated focus, albeit on a larger scale and in different services, is similar to that of for-profit firms. Secular nonprofit and public providers in contrast offer a much more comprehensive set of services.

Providers also differ in their approaches within service categories. FBOs provide a strong and unique emphasis on transitional assistance– the only provider type that focuses on such interventions. Within mental health services, we find evidence that different providers emphasize different means of delivery, and that these differences are consistent with their resources and missions.

Thus, the results delineate a complementary role for FBOs in the provision of social services, through their emphasis on transitional assistance, their multi-service orientation, and their reliance on interventions that utilize their unique strengths. Faith-based organizations do not represent a substitute for secular providers. Both in terms of quantity and breadth of service offerings, secular nonprofits and public providers dominate social service delivery.

These results, of course, may be unique to the community studied. Los Angeles County is far from typical on any measure of urban environments. It is larger, more ethnically diverse, and faces exaggerated challenges compared to most other urban communities. Many such community-based studies need to be conducted and compared on the types of evaluative criteria developed here. Developing this body of knowledge offers the most promising approach for increasing our understanding of the roles different types of service providers play in the delivery of social services, and helping us develop reasonable expectations about the specific role that can be played by faith-based organizations.

NOTES

1. INFOLINE of Los Angeles is a private nonprofit provider of human services information and referrals. It is the largest, most technologically advanced referral service in the nation, serving 200,000 people per year. We thank Susan Brown Campbell for generously providing access to these data.

2. INFOLINE defines human services as programs addressing "human needs ranging from basic living needs such as food and shelter through life improvement services such as education, to life enhancement programs such as cultural programs." (INFOLINE Inclusion Criteria)

3. Kearns, Park, and Yankoski (2005) also studied a broad set of self-defined faith-based community service providers in Pittsburgh, and compared them with secular nonprofit providers. They found little difference in size, funding, self-reported organizational capacity, and management sophistication between the two groups. This comparability in organizational characteristics provides additional support for the need to look beyond the behavior of congregations in understanding faith-based service delivery.

4. The original data set included services provided by out-of-county agencies, by agencies with no identified ownership type, and by 13 coalitions of unspecified ownership. These were deleted to create the data set analyzed in this study.

5. There is an on-going effort in the literature to more carefully define the term "faith-based" to enhance its analytic usefulness (e.g., Smith and Sosin, 2001; Jeavons, 2003; Sider and Unruh, 2004). Such efforts will improve our ability to differentiate expected behavior *within* this organizational category.

6. Note that these data do not indicate size of effort. So they do not reveal any information about how many service recipients are aided by the different type of providers.

7. This is consistent with Twombly (2002)'s findings about differences in funding across secular and religious social service organizations.

REFERENCES

Anderson, S.D., Orr, J., & Silverman, C. (2000). *Can we make welfare reform work? The California religious community capacity study.* Sacramento, CA: The California Council of Churches.

Bartkowski, J.P., & Regis, H.A. (1999). *Religious organizations, anti-poverty relief and Charitable Choice: A feasibility study of faith-based welfare reform in Mississippi.* Arlington, VA: PricewaterhouseCoopers, Endowment for the Business of Government.

Botchwey, N.D.S. (2003). *Taxonomy of religious and secular nonprofit organizations: Knowledge development and policy recommendations for neighborhood revitalization.* Unpublished doctoral dissertation. Philadelphia: University of Pennsylvania, Department of City and Regional Planning.

Center for Public Justice. (1997). *A guide to Charitable Choice: The rules of section 104 of the 1996 federal welfare law governing state cooperation with faith-based social-service providers.* Washington, DC: Center for Public Justice.

Chaves, M. (1999). Religious congregations and welfare reform: Who will take advantage of Charitable Choice? *American Sociological Review, 64* (December), 836-846.

_____, & Tsitsos, W. (2001). Congregations and social services: What they do, how they do it, and with whom. *Nonprofit and Voluntary Sector Quarterly,* 30, 660-683.

Cnaan, R. (1999). Our hidden safety net: Social & community work by urban American religious congregations. *Brookings Review,* 17 (2), 50-53.

_____, & Boddie, S. (2001). Philadelphia census of congregations and their involvement in social service delivery. *The Social Service Review,* 75 (4), 559-581.

Etindi, D. (1999). Charitable Choice and its implications for faith-based organizations. *The Welfare Reformer,* 1 (1). Washington, DC: Hudson, Institute, Welfare Policy Center.

Grettenberger, S.E. (2000). *The role of churches in non-religious services: United Methodist Churches in Michigan.* Working Paper. Washington, DC: The Aspen Institute Nonprofit Sector Research Fund.

Griener, G. (2000). Charitable Choice and welfare reform: Collaboration between state and local governments and faith-based organizations. *Welfare Information Network Issue Notes,* 4 (September).

Jeavons, T.H. (2003). The vitality and independence of religious organizations. *Society,* 40 (2), 27-36.

Kearns, K., Park, C., & Yankowski, L. (2005). Comparing faith-based and secular community service corporations in Pittsburgh and Allegheny County, Pennsylvania. *Nonprofit and Voluntary Sector Quarterly,* 34 (2), 206-31.

Kennedy, S.S., & Bielefeld, W. (2002). Government shekels without government shackles: The administrative challenges of Charitable Choice. *Public Administrative Review, 62* (January/February), 4-11.

Los Angeles County Department of Health Services. (1999). *L.A. health profiles.* Los Angeles, CA: Los Angeles County Department of Health Services, Office of Health Assessment and Epidemiology.

Printz, T.J. (1998). Faith-based service providers in the nation's capital: Can they do more? *Charting Civil Society,* 2 (April). Washington, DC: The Urban Institute, Center on Nonprofits and Philanthropy.

Sherman, A.L. (2000). *The growing impact of Charitable Choice: A catalogue of new collaborations between government and faith-based organizations in nine states.* Washington, DC: Center for Public Justice.

Sider, R.J., & Unruh, H.R. (2004). Typology of religious characteristics of social service and educational organizations and programs. *Nonprofit and Voluntary Sector Quarterly,* 33 (1), 109-134.

Smith, S.R., & Sosin, M.R. (2001). The varieties of faith-related agencies. *Public Administration Review, 61* (November/December), 651-670.

Trulear, H.D. (2000). Faith-based institutions and high-risk youth. *Field Report Series, (Spring).* Philadelphia, PA: Public/Private Ventures.

Twombly, E.C. (2002). Religious versus secular human service organizations: Implications for public policy. *Social Science Quarterly,* 83(4), 947-961.

Wolpert, J., & Seley, J. E., with Motta-Moss, A. (2004). *Nonprofit services in New York City's neighborhoods: An analysis of access, responsiveness, and coverage.* New York City Nonprofits Project.

Yates, J. (1998). Partnerships with the faith community in welfare reform. *Welfare Information Network Issue Notes,* 2 (March).

APPENDIX
Service Categories

Arts & Culture (cultural awareness, fine and performing arts programs, interpreter and translator services)

Business Services (business services, check cashing outlets, farmers' markets, thrift shops)

Civil Rights (advocacy, human rights)

Community Improvement (community action groups, community relations, community services, planning and zoning)

Education (K-12, vocational/technical, higher education, adult/continuing, libraries, literacy programs, education services, post-secondary education, professional education, school districts, special education, family life education, student services & organizations)

Environment & Animals (conservation, environmental services, flood control, garden services, trash collection and disposal, animal-related services)

Food (food service/distribution, nutrition promotion, home economics, congregate meals, emergency food, food services, home delivered meals, senior nutrition programs, summer food service program)

General Health (hospitals/clinics, outpatient, reproductive health, health support services, emergency medical services, public health & wellness, health care financing/insurance, nursing)

*Housing/Shelter (*housing, temporary, homeless, support services, bad weather shelter, housing services, shelter, transitional shelter)

Jobs (vocational training, employment procurement assistance, vocational rehab, labor unions, labor-management)

Mental Health (alcohol, drug, substance abuse prevention & treatment, addiction, mental health, psychiatric care, counseling)

Other Human Services (multipurpose human services, children & youth services, family services, financial counseling, emergency assistance)

Philanthropy & Voluntarism (voluntarism promotion)

Public Protection (police & law enforcement, correctional facilities & prisoner services, crime/violence prevention, rehabilitation of offenders, courts & justice administration, dispute/conflict resolution, protection against abuse–child, sexual, spouse, legal services)

Public Safety (building and safety, disaster services, fire and rescue services, first aid & safety programs)

Public/Society Benefit (benefits programs, consumer services, public awareness/education, public works, services to military personnel, tax assistance, utilities, veterans' benefits)

Recreation (Parks, recreational programs)

Youth Development (youth centers, Big Brothers/Sisters, citizenship, residential care, services for seniors, women, homeless, etc.)

Chapter 8

Investigating the Implementation of Charitable Choice

Wolfgang Bielefeld

SUMMARY. This paper reports on a project to investigate the implementation of charitable choice in TANF-funded job services in Indiana, Massachusetts, and North Carolina. A number of issues needed to be addressed in the course of the research project. State-level government responses to charitable choice were found to vary widely, making comparisons across states difficult. In Indiana, job training providers and clients were also interviewed. For providers, a major research issue was the assessment of the degree to which they were faith-based and the impact of this. To measure the impact of provider faith orientation on clients, a pre- and post-service study was designed. Providers were to administer the tests, but in many cases failed to do so correctly, thereby limiting the utility of the results. Finally, during the last year of the study, the state changed its funding priorities, thereby altering the provider system. A number of the providers changed their programs or stopped providing services, thereby dropping out of the delivery system. The paper considers

Wolfgang Bielefeld, PhD, is affiliated with School of Public and Environmental Affairs, Indiana University–Purdue University Indianapolis (E-mail: wbielefe@iupui. edu).

The author wishes to thank the editors for helpful feedback received during the writing of this paper.

Funding for this project was provided by a grant from the Ford Foundation.

[Haworth co-indexing entry note]: "Investigating the Implementation of Charitable Choice." Bielefeld, Wolfgang. Co-published simultaneously in *Journal of Religion & Spirituality in Social Work* (The Haworth Pastoral Press, an imprint of The Haworth Press, Inc.) Vol. 25, No. 3/4, 2006, pp. 151-173; and: *Faith-Based Social Services: Measures, Assessments, and Effectiveness* (ed: Stephanie C. Boddie, and Ram A. Cnaan) The Haworth Pastoral Press, an imprint of The Haworth Press, Inc., 2006, pp. 151-173.

the impact of these difficulties on the ability of research to make contributions to the discussion of charitable choice.

KEYWORDS. Charitable choice, faith-based service providers, program implementation, program evaluation

In 2000, a three-year research project was launched to study the implementation of charitable choice in Indiana, Massachusetts, and North Carolina. Given the contentious nature of the public debate associated with and the significant issues raised by charitable choice, it is important to assess the impacts of this policy initiative. These assessments will not be easy, however. This paper discusses the challenges that researchers in one project encountered as they sought to do so.

One of the more controversial elements of recent welfare reform is the charitable choice provision. Charitable choice, or Section 104 of the Personal Responsibility and Work Opportunity Reconciliation Act of 1996 (PRWORA), encourages states to contract with faith-based organizations (FBOs) for the delivery of social services to welfare recipients on the same basis used to contract with traditional, secular providers. Charitable choice, as conceived in 1996, allows faith-based service providers to use religious criteria when hiring staff, to maintain religious symbols in areas where programs are administered, and to use faith-based concepts when providing services. Clients have a right to an alternative secular provider and may not be pressured or forced to participate in religious observances. Public funds may not be used for sectarian activities such as worship, religious instruction, or proselytizing.

Historically, significant funds have gone to social service providers who were affiliated with and informed by the religious precepts of FBOs, and government funds have followed individual hospital patients and nursing home residents to religious facilities. However, charitable choice initiatives go further and encourage governments to partner directly with sectarian organizations–including organizations considered "pervasively sectarian"–in order to provide an array of social services.

There has been a sustained discussion of the pros and cons of service provision by FBOs since the passage of charitable choice. Proponents of charitable choice opened the debate with claims about the benefits that faith-based service providers would bring to social service delivery systems. On the macro level, they hold that including FBOs will increase the diversity in delivery systems, thereby enhancing government responsiveness (Wilson, 2003). The proponents also claim that FBOs are more efficient and that the services they provide are more effective (see Sherman, 2003, and White House, 2001 for summaries). In terms of efficiency, FBOs may have access to infrastructures, volunteers, and existing community networks that can be used for service provision (either directly by a congregation or via a separate 501(c)(3)). They are also likely to be smaller and, therefore, less bureaucratic. With their reliance on faith, these providers may provide a "better" service than their secular counterparts. They may be more holistic in their approach to individual clients, and therefore promote the transformation of clients in ways secular organizations do not. They also may establish more personal, caring, and enduring relationships with clients than do secular providers (their services may be more likely to include mentoring, role models, and ongoing support networks). They may have more motivated staff, access to motivated volunteers, and existing networks that enhance their reach into the community and enhance the scope of their service delivery.

Those who are skeptical about charitable choice have argued that government support of FBOs may erode the separation of church and state; may promote employment discrimination; and may, in fact, result in favoritism for faith-based providers (Chaves, 2003). In addition, conclusive evidence that faith-based providers (either congregations or the 501(c)(3)s affiliated with them) perform better, or even differently, on the whole than secular providers has not been presented (Chaves, 2003; Johnson, Tompkins, & Webb, 2002; United States General Accounting Office, 2002).

In order to shed light on the workings of service delivery systems containing FBOs, a three-year research project, funded by the Ford Foundation, was launched in 2000 at the School for Public and Environmental Affairs at Indiana University–Purdue University Indianapolis. The project examined the implementation of charitable choice in Indiana, Massachusetts, and North Carolina. The project compared these state's use of FBOs to provide job training services funded by the Temporary Assistance to Needy Families program (TANF). The project sought to assess:

1. Differences in state implementation approaches to charitable choice
2. The organizational characteristics, capacities, and effectiveness of providers
3. The attitudinal and behavioral impacts on clients of faith-based providers

It quickly became apparent that a series of conceptual and methodological issues needed to be addressed over the course of the research and during the interpretation of the findings. These included issues that surfaced at both the state and local level.

ACROSS-STATE CULTURAL DIFFERENCES

In the American federalist system, the form and impacts of federal-level initiatives will be significantly shaped and moderated by factors at the state level. Legislation, mandates, and programs originating in Washington are likely to end up taking a variety of forms by the time they end up "on the ground" in the fifty states. A plethora of political, economic, and social factors can affect state implementation efforts, ranging from relatively straight-forward conditions such as the state's wealth or poverty to cultural factors such as the values and attitudes of the majority of the state's residents. The results of charitable choice implementation in a given state will depend, therefore, upon a host of factors specific to that state. To illustrate the differences in charitable choice implementation between states, we chose three states for our study. They vary on political culture, a dimension which we felt was important for determining how charitable choice would be delivered at the local level.

For our purposes, we relied upon the theoretical and descriptive analysis of political culture provided by Daniel Elazar (1994). Elazar defines political culture as a multi-faceted concept; specifically, "the particular pattern of orientation to political action in which each political system is embedded" (1984, p. 109). Through the analysis of movements of early American immigrant populations with distinctive political cultures over the course of the country's settlement, he established a relationship between public attitudes and various political dimensions, including orientation toward bureaucracy, views about government intervention in private affairs and program initiation, popular participation in elections, and the importance attached to political parties. The dimensions serve as criteria for classifying states and substate areas today according to three types of political culture–moralistic, traditionalistic, and individualistic. Each state and locality is classified as purely moralistic, purely traditionalistic, purely individualistic, or a combination of any two.

One of Elazar's dimensions, the role of government in society, is central to the theme of this paper. Citizens in an individualistic culture prefer a government that functions primarily "to keep the marketplace in proper working order" (1986, p. 173). An individualistic culture emphasizes the centrality of private concerns, looks askance at most government interventions, and sees political activity in quite "transactional" terms. According to Elazar's typological map (1986, p. 177) the middle and western states are oriented toward individualism. Citizens in a moralistic culture, on the other hand, have a "commonwealth conception" (1972, p. 96) of democracy. Government, in this view, is a positive means to promote the public welfare and holding political office is viewed as a public service. This culture is prevalent in New England and in Northern plains states such as Wisconsin and Minnesota. Finally, the traditionalistic culture, which Elazar describes as paternalistic and elitist, is characterized by the view that government's principal role is to maintain elitist dominance of the "existing social order" (1972, p. 99). It functions to confine power to a relatively small group of people, and one's place in the power structure is determined through family and other ties to the elite. In traditionalistic cultures, political systems tend to be dominated by a single party, and political leaders play a "conservative and custodial" role. This culture is found predominantly in the South.

According to Elazar's political culture map, Massachusetts is shown as primarily moralistic, Indiana is virtually all individualistic, and North Carolina is predominantly traditionalistic. The three states, therefore, reflected one of the three political cultures and these differences can be expected to influence the ways in which the states approached the implementation of charitable choice. In his study of the effect of political culture on PRWORA implementation generally, Lawrence Mead also referred to the Elazar categories, summarizing them as follows:

> Moralistic politics stresses problem solving, not partisan rivalry. In the individualistic style, goals are less high-minded, but there is also more tolerance for disagreement, and often more willingness

to compromise. Both moralistic and individualistic states tend to have well-developed bureaucracies. In the traditionalistic style, social policymaking and administration are less well developed. (Mead, 2004)

Mead also analyzed state implementation of PRWORA, looking at both political and administrative performance. Mead found significant differences among the states that correlated to Elazar's political culture categories. Those differences were consistent with the charitable choice implementation differences we observed.

Looking at developments since 1996 in Indiana, Massachusetts, and North Carolina, we discovered dramatically different reactions to Section 104.[1] For each of these different states, we asked a series of common questions about the contracting culture of the state and the interpretation and implementation of charitable choice. We found that Massachusetts was essentially unmoved by the enactment of Section 104. In the seven years that the provision has been Federal law, the Commonwealth has done almost nothing to alter the conditions under which religious organizations compete for purchase of service contracts or operate publicly funded welfare programs (Jensen, 2003). Massachusetts approached charitable choice pragmatically, with a minimum of partisan rivalry. Elected and appointed officials analyzed the statutory language, determined the criteria to be employed, and concluded that the state was in compliance.

Both Indiana and North Carolina responded more actively to the charitable choice. Their responses, however, differed markedly. In Indiana, there also was little partisanship involved in implementation. The Democratic administration decided to embrace charitable choice, but–in a spirit of compromise characteristic of individualistic cultures–limited the state's involvement to job training and placement programs, services unlikely to implicate constitutional issues or passions. Outreach in Indiana was consistently framed in classic individualist terms: the interim Director of Family and Social Service Administration explained that the state was open to any contractor, secular or religious, who could do the job. In North Carolina, where policymaking "appeared to be casual and personalized,"(Mead, 2004: 282), and where government has historically had difficulty recruiting capable people, reflecting "the low prestige and low pay of public service in traditionalistic cultures" (Mead, 2004: 284), implementation efforts occurred largely outside state government, either through pilot projects funded by the state but managed by nonprofit agencies, or in response to initiatives of religious organizations themselves.

These findings have implications for how local delivery systems in these, or any, states can be compared. Political culture, like many other factors, sets parameters within which state implementation efforts take place. These need to be considered in the comparison of implementation efforts. For example, is charitable choice, as promoted by the Bush administration, more compatible with any of the three political cultures as they are manifest in the three states under study? If so, to what degree has this influenced state implementation of charitable choice? The answers are not clear. Charitable choice seems to embody a combination of individualistic and moralistic political culture elements, seeking at the same time to promote enhanced competition between private sector actors (an individualistic orientation element) as well as the direction and use of public funds to promote community welfare and values (a moralistic orientation element). In any case, detailed local-level comparative research would be needed to assess the degree to which a political culture which was compatible with these federal ends would influence state implementation efforts and shape local delivery systems. This comparative research could also examine the relationship between charitable choice, state political culture and religious factors. For example, is state political culture associated with the prevalence of any particular faith orientations in the state and does this have any relation to the types of services provided, types of clients served, or client outcomes of religious versus secular providers in the state? Further, if these types of relationships are found, how might they influence the implementation of charitable choice in a state?

Unfortunately, the research project did not have the resources to carry out three detailed comparative local studies of the kind suggested above. Consequently, the specific ramifications for local services of state-level political culture differences could not be assessed. The project was, however, able to study the local delivery system in one state–Indiana. This was due primarily to the fact that the research team was headquartered there. Indiana, never-the-less, has been the one of the most active proponents of charitable choice, making it a good subject for more detailed study. The fact that Indiana has an individualistic political culture, might also lead to the hypothesis that this political culture is the most compatible with charitable choice. Future studies, however, will be needed to address this hypothesis in a systematic fashion. In any case, while not having to deal with the issues of comparative research raised above, the examination of the Indiana delivery system uncovered a host of other issues unique to the local level.

LOCAL DELIVERY SYSTEMS ISSUES

The Indiana Provider Study

Our analysis of Indiana providers focused specifically on the Indiana Manpower Placement and Comprehensive Training program (IMPACT). IMPACT is funded by the Temporary Assistance for Needy Families (TANF) block grant, administered by Indiana's Family Social Service Administration. IMPACT funds employment-based services including assessment; education; job training; job readiness; and job search, development, and placement. IMPACT contracts with newly formed and traditional faith-based providers as well as with non-faith-based providers to deliver these services. Client and provider relations are handled by county welfare departments. In our research, we assessed the operations of local providers, impacts on client's attitudes and religious behavior, and changes in the delivery system over time. We encountered significant challenges in each portion of the research. For providers, a major issue was measuring the degree to which religion influenced their operations. For client impacts, administering the pre- and post-service study design proved problematic. Finally, the delivery system changed in the final year of the study, making comparisons between years difficult.

The IMPACT Delivery System

To assess provider operations, we conducted interviews in person and by mail with IMPACT provider administrators in 2001 and 2002 to assess a variety of operational factors. We designed the provider questionnaire to gather data on factors deemed important for assessing the efficacy of service provision. We developed these factors and the questionnaire from the literature and conference presentations on organizational structure and process, charitable choice and faith-based service provision, and from other ongoing nonprofit surveys.

The questionnaire asked about basic organizational factors such as revenue, IMPACT contract amounts, and the number of agency and

IMPACT employees and volunteers. One of our key goals was to measure the degree to which faith influences the providers. To do this, we developed a series of questions and constructed a faith-influence scale, described in more detail below. If an organization was determined to be faith-based on this scale, we asked the respondent a series of questions about the consequences of this orientation. In addition, we used a set of questions about the types of services provided by the organization to assess the degree to which the organization has a holistic orientation toward its clients. We measured organizational involvement in networks by formal affiliation, IMPACT-related contacts, and community involvements. We also categorized the purpose of these links. In addition, we measured the degree to which clients came from the immediate neighborhood. Finally we assessed the degree to which providers reported management challenges on key factors associated with governance, internal operations, and external relations.

For this project, we attempted to interview all providers from three Indiana counties (Lake, Marion, and Miami). In each of these counties, some of the IMPACT providers had been designated by the state as "faith-based" based on either (1) their participation in a program designed to reach out to FBOs by providing technical assistance and capacity building (FaithWorks), or (2) their self-identification as faith-based.

We found that there were 34 IMPACT providers in the three counties. We obtained interviews with 30 of these: 3 in Miami County, 13 in Lake County, and 14 in Marion County. The interviewed providers included 22 nonprofits, 5 for-profits, and 3 government agencies. One nonprofit and three for-profit IMPACT providers did not agree to be interviewed.

Measuring the Influence of Faith

In research on FBOs, a major issue is how to define the term "faith-based" (Chambre, 2001; Jeavons, 1998; Search for Common Ground, 2002; and Smith & Sosin, 2001). The state of Indiana classifies providers as faith-based or not depending on two factors: self-identification (the chief method) and/or participation in the FaithWorks program. This simple binary distinction is inadequate, and numerous researchers have pointed out that it is more useful to think of the degree of religiosity as a dimension (Green & Sherman, 2002; Jeavons, 1998; Monsma & Mounts, 2002; Search for Common Ground, 2002; Smith et al., 2001). Table 1 compares the dimensions included by several re-

TABLE 1. A Comparison of Dimensions and Indicators Used in Identification of Faith-Based Organizations

Dimensions and Indicators	Jeavons 1998	Smith & Sosin (2001)	Finding Common Ground (2002)	Green & Sherman (2002)	Monsma & Mounts (2002)	Bielefeld, Littlepage & Thelin (2002)
Formal/Informal Religious Affiliation						
Religious name	X					
Religious authority coupling		X				
Affiliated with religious agency			X			X
Founded by religious organization			X			
Religion in Mission/Governance						
Mission statement is explicitly religious			X	X		
Establishing separate 501(c)(3) would be a problem			X			
Religious criteria for board	X		X	X		
Senior management/other staff share faith	X		X	X	X	X
Religion in Funding						
Financial Support/ Resource dependency	X	X	X			X
Receives reimbursement for providing "entitlement" services			X			
Religion in Structure and/or Process						
Percent of participants in organization holding religious conviction	X					
Religious culture		X				
Religious symbols or pictures			X		X	X
Opening or closing sessions with prayer					X	X (meals)
Prayer or texts guide decisions	X					X
Faith criteria used to assign staff	X			X	X	X
Uses religious values to motivate staff					X	
Partners with religious organizations	X					

Dimensions and Indicators	Jeavons 1998	Smith & Sosin (2001)	Finding Common Ground (2002)	Green & Sherman (2002)	Monsma & Mounts (2002)	Bielefeld, Littlepage & Thelin (2002)
Religion in Services to Clients						
Religion or faith is a part of services	X		X	X		X
Voluntary religious exercises for clients				X	X	X
Requires religious exercises for clients					X	X
Uses religious values to encourage attitude change			X	X	X	
Encourages clients to make religious commitments				X	X	X
Gives preference to clients who are in religious agreement				X	X	X

searchers in their classifications of the degree to which faith influences service providers.

Based on this previous work, especially Jeavons, we asked our respondents six screening questions about the influence of faith on their organization (the first six dimensions shown in Table 2). As expected, we found variations in the degree to which faith influenced the providers.

Of the 30 providers surveyed, 17 had no affirmative responses to the screening questions. We consider these not influenced at all by faith or religion and designated them as non-faith-based (NFB) providers. We consider the remaining 13 organizations faith-based and gave them one point for each affirmative response to the six screening questions. The faith-based organizations were then given a series of follow-up questions to measure two additional dimensions–visible religiousness and implicit religiousness (the last two rows in Table 2). An organization was given a point if they answered "yes" to any of the questions in the visible dimension group and a point if they answered "yes" to any of the questions in the implicit dimension group. Our scale, therefore, could range from zero to eight.

We categorized organizations that had one to four points as moderately faith-based (MFB) and organizations with more than four points as strongly faith-based (SFB). Of those found to be influenced by faith,

TABLE 2. Dimensions Used in Measuring the Influence of Faith

Dimension	Question
Funding	Organization provides funds or support to any religious organizations
Affiliation	Organization affiliated with any religious organizations or faith traditions
Shared Belief	Desired, requested, or required that staff and volunteers share the same religious belief or faith
Services	Religion or faith part of any services provided
Decision Making	Organizational decisions guided by prayer or religious texts, documents, or periodicals
Staff Assignment	Religious or faith criteria used to assign staff to positions
Visible Religiousness	Yes to any of these: religious leader on staff, efforts to encourage clients to make personal religious commitments, required religious exercises, and spoken prayers at meals
Implicit Religiousness	Yes to any of these: religious symbols/pictures in the facility, generalized spirit of love among staff, voluntary religious exercises, informal references to religious ideas by staff to clients, and staff that are members of the congregation

six were found to be MFB and seven SFB. As Table 3 indicates, four of the for-profit providers were faith-based. We had not expected to find FBOs operating under this auspice and their status was only revealed during the interviews. As far as we know, this type of provider has not been identified nor their operations examined in the literature on charitable choice. In his study, Monsma (2004) identified a number of for-profits which provided welfare-to-work services. These, however, were assigned to a separate category in his analysis and their faith orientation is not discussed. So, while it is not clear if these for-profits were faith-based or not, the implication is that they were secular in orientation.

The technique we used raises a number of issues. In the first place, it should be noted that our categorization of faith influence depends on the current director's practices and perceptions of the organization. The categorization could change if leadership changes. An example of this is that one provider with a historic religious affiliation and several locations in Indiana was categorized as MFB at one location, but as NFB at another location. Also, we only interviewed top management and,

TABLE 3. Faith Orientation of IMPACT Providers by Type or Organization

Type of Organization	Faith Influence*	Number of Organizations	Average Age of Organization (years)	Average Number of Full-Time Employees
Nonprofit	NFB	13	37	39
	MFB	3	64	292
	SFB	6	10	2
	Total	22	33	63
For-profit	NFB	1	6	20
	MFB	3	3	5
	SFB	1	23	1
	Total	5	8	7
Government Agency	NFB	3	62	250
	MFB	0		
	SFB	0		
	Total	3	62	250
Grand Total		30	62	126

*Note: NFB = Non-Faith-Based (Score of 0 on Faith Influence Questions)
   MFB = Moderately Faith-Based (Score of 1-4 on Faith Influence Questions
   SFB = Strongly Faith-Based (Score of 5-7 on Faith Influence Questions)

sometimes, program supervisors. Cost factors prohibited us from interviewing front line service-providing staff. It is important, however, to assess client-service staff interactions to get an idea of how faith does or does not "work." But, even interviews at this level may not be enough, given differences in ideas about what using religion in service delivery entails. This means that observational methods will likely be needed to provide the most valid information. This will be discussed further in the section on client impacts.

Faith and the Operation of Providers

As we outlined in the introduction, proponents of charitable choice often portray faith-based organizations as more holistic, more connected to their community, able to make better use of volunteers, and more community-based than secular providers. The results of our interviews with this small sample of providers in Indiana shed light on their involvement in one service delivery system. Only a short summary will be presented here; further details can be found in Bielefeld, Littlepage, and Thelin (2003).

Our findings are mixed. Our results show that, in this delivery system, the SFB providers are small, have smaller IMPACT contracts, and are more reliant on these contracts for revenue. Religion is more prevalent in SFB providers, they feel comfortable in their use of religion in services, they have more clients who participated in religious activity, but have more negative issues about religion with clients. When asked what issues clients have had with religious-based practices, one SFB provider said that one client was Muslim and other students' faiths made her uncomfortable (although she stayed with the program). Another SFB said that some clients left because they did not want to be in a church. We found only a slight (and negative) relation between faith influence and the holistic nature of service provision. SFB providers, were, however, more likely to provide non-IMPACT services for which they were not reimbursed. When we examined their networks, the SFB organizations seem to be the somewhat less connected than the MFB organizations. Given their small size, however, their average number of links that SFB providers have is noteworthy. We also found that for SFB providers, their involvement with IMPACT leads to more other community involvements (thereby enlarging their networks) and changed their relations with other organizations. They are also less likely to use volunteers, but when they do use volunteers, they are more likely to use them to provide IMPACT services. This may be one way they compensate for their smaller staff size. Finally, SFB providers seem to focus their services more on their immediate neighborhood. The SFB provider's tighter geographic service area may be a reflection of smaller size or possibly an intentional neighborhood focus.

The FBOs in our study have, according to our questions, management strengths and weaknesses. More strongly faith-based providers indicated greater challenges mostly in the areas of governance and external relations. The former include recruiting and keeping effective board members and managing board/staff relations. The latter include strategic planning and delivering high quality services. They also had more challenges with internal operations in terms of managing facilities. A number of these challenges were also related to age or size. On the other hand, more strongly faith-based providers reported fewer challenges with mission accomplishment and a number of internal processes including internal communication, internal working relationships, anticipating financial needs, obtaining funding, using technology for service provision, recruiting/keeping qualified administrators, and managing programs. None of these was related to size and only the last was related to age.

When we examined differences between MFB nonprofit and for-profit providers, a number of findings emerged. The MFB for-profit providers were more reliant on their IMPACT contracts for revenue. They were less likely to be formally affiliated or otherwise linked with other organizations and their relations to other organizations did not change due to their IMPACT contract. Finally, they were less likely to use volunteers and none of them uses volunteers to provide IMPACT services. Our comparison of non and for-profit providers also indicates that the for-profits reported fewer management challenges than the nonprofits in every faith orientation category. For MFB providers, non- and for-profits were similar in regard to governance/mission and external relations. For-profits, however, indicated fewer problems with internal operations. We could speculate that in the for-profits, a more explicit recognition or acknowledgement of a need or desire to make a profit might give management an added incentive and rationale to focus internal operations.

Client Attitudinal and Behavioral Outcomes

In previous studies, one factor that has not been examined directly is the perspective of and the impact on the clients receiving social services from faith-based providers. This is an important oversight, since FBOs, with their reliance on faith, have been purported to provide a "better" service than their secular counterparts. They are said to be more holistic in their approach to individual clients and therefore promote the transformation of clients in ways secular organizations do not. This suggests the existence of an intervening variable that can be conceptualized as personal transformation. Do clients of faith-based providers become more "religious?" Do faith-based providers impact more of the "whole" person–improving self-image and making them feel better about themselves? There is a large body of literature in the health field that documents the effects of religion and spirituality on well-being and self-esteem (Johnson et al., 2002; McCullough, Hoyt, Larson, Koenig, & Thoresen, 2000).

THE PROGRAM OUTCOME SURVEY

We designed a pre- and post-service study to shed light on this question. Further details about the study can be found in Littlepage, Thelin, Bielefeld, and Sedaca (2003). Clients were to receive a short survey at the start of their services and another when they completed their program. As clients started and finished programs at various times, the providers were to give them the surveys at the appropriate points. Providers were given the surveys, self-addressed envelopes to return them to us, and modest grocery store vouchers to give to their clients when they completed either the pre- or the post-survey. Clients were to indicate their initials on the surveys, which would allow us to match pre- and post-surveys.

Surveys were distributed in this way to clients of three of the faith-based providers and three of the NFB providers who agreed to participate in this phase of the study. While we received surveys from all the participating providers, many of the surveys we received were not usable. We received pre-surveys from 152 clients but usable pre- and post-surveys from only 60 clients. Surveys were unusable for a number of reasons, all having to do with improper administration by providers. In some cases, both pre- and post-surveys were administered on the same day. In other cases, pre-surveys were given to participants who had been in the program for several months or the post-surveys were never administered. It is possible that these administrative errors occurred by mistake. On the other hand, they could have occurred so that providers could give their clients as many food vouchers as possible, thereby providing a benefit for their clients. In any case, this resulted in usable pre- and post-surveys from two faith-based providers and three non-faith-based providers. The data consists of responses from 37 clients for NFB providers, 14 clients from a MFB provider and 9 clients from a SFB provider.

The characteristics of the clients whose responses we could use, on the whole, mirrored those of the total group of clients in the project. Roughly half of the responding clients had a high school diploma or GED certificate, a percentage similar to the total client group (52 percent). We should note, though, that none of the responding clients from the SFB provider had post-high school education, whereas seven percent of the total client group did. In addition, approximately 80 percent of the responding clients were female and about 80 percent were non-white. Both of these percentages were similar to the total client group.

Was Religion a Part of Services?

In the post-service survey we asked if religion was a part of the services received. For each type of provider, a portion of their clients felt that religion was a part of the IMPACT services they received; including (interestingly) 12 percent of NFB clients, 17 percent of MFB clients, and 11 percent of SFB clients. We found, moreover, that another portion of the clients in each type of provider reported that they were "unsure" about whether religion was or was not a part of the services they received. This included 12 percent of NFB clients, 17 percent of MFB clients, and 44 percent of SFB clients.

This uncertainty may be attributable to clients' awareness that while the IMPACT services are being offered on religious premises and sometimes by a religious leader, the providers try to offer IMPACT services that are free of religion. It also could be related to a client's doubt as to what is meant by "religion" in the context of service provision. In one case, for example, the research team observed a class being taught during which the instructor relayed information about their own salvation. Later in the class, one of the students became distraught and the student and teacher left the classroom for a short time in order to pray together. In a focus group discussion afterwards, the students were asked if religion was part of the class. They responded that is was not. In any case, all clients who perceived religion as part of IMPACT services thought it was helpful to them and felt comfortable with it, including those in NFBs.

This does, though, bring up the issue of how to measure the religiosity of services with surveys if clients themselves are unsure. For instance, for some clients the expression of religious conviction may be such an integral part of everyday life that the inclusion of such expressions of faith in service provision is not seen as anything noteworthy or special. Other clients, however, may perceive and label these expressions of faith delivered in service provision as religiously-oriented services. This reinforces the point made earlier about the necessity of gathering observational/subjective data in addition to survey/objective data.

Did Clients Change?

In both the pre- and post-service surveys we asked about the client's participation in religious services, praying, and reading religious texts. We also asked about perceived level of control in personal life, and

self-image. Clients of the three types of providers report similar perceptions of self-image. The majority of clients of each provider type indicate high levels of self-assurance on the pre-service surveys and the
changes between surveys were roughly equal in positive and negative
directions.

Table 4 shows percentages and changes for the religious behavior
items. The table shows that the clients of MFB providers were the most
religious at the start of their services, while the clients of SFB increased
their religious behavior the most on two of the items. In terms of the frequency of attending religious services, SFB clients were least likely to
do so at the start. They did show small increases by the end of their services. These were, however, comparable to the changes for NFB provider clients. For praying privately and reading religious material,
however, SFB clients, while roughly similar to NFB clients at the start
of their services, increased their behavior to a far greater degree than
their NFB counterparts.

While the sample size is small and the administration of the surveys
leaves much to be desired, the results are intriguing and suggest that the
SFB providers did have an influence on some dimensions of their cli-

TABLE 4. Client Reports of Religious Behavior–Pre- and Post-Surveys

Provider Faith Orientation	% Clients with Frequent Behavior (Pre-Test)*	% Clients Increasing Behavior (Post-Test)
Attendance at Religious Services		
NFB	49%	14%
MFB	71%	0
SFB	12%	11%
Praying Privately		
NFB	54%	27%
MFB	86%	14%
SFB	56%	44%
Reading Religious Material		
NFB	10%	3%
MFB	31%	7%
SFB	22%	22%

* Religious Services: frequently = at least 2 or 3 times a month
Praying privately and reading religious material: frequently = once or more a day

ent's religious behavior. Many questions remain to be answered on the durability and consequences of this behavior, of course.

Delivery System Changes

In Indiana, there was a concerted effort to expand FBO participation in IMPACT, with a consequent modest increase in participation by FBOs. This was short-lived, however, as the state experienced budget problems and both cut back IMPACT funding and changed the program's priorities. These had significant effects on the delivery system and made comparison of the program in 2001 and 2003 problematic. A summary of this is provided below and further details can be found in Thelin (2003).

Beginning in 1998, the state has been aggressive in its outreach and education to FBOs and the faith community. In 1999, the state requested applications for a contractor to administer a technical assistance program aimed at recruiting and educating FBOs, to be called FaithWorks. Among the goals of the initiative were outreach to the faith community, development of technical assistance materials and a training program, and efforts to increase awareness of charitable choice in the faith community. A for-profit consulting firm (one of three applicants), was selected for a two-year $500,000 contract. The contract was subsequently extended for a third year, through November 2002.

In 2000, roughly 75 of 400 groups (both faith-based and non-faith-based) who had attended a FaithWorks technical assistance workshop applied for state contracts. About 40 contracts were subsequently awarded to faith-based groups in a variety of programs (using the state definition for a faith-based organization–self-identification, and participation in FaithWorks). Data shows that the number of faith-based providers in the IMPACT program increased during contract years 2000 and 2001–growing from three to nine. In contract year 2002, however, the number of faith–based providers dropped to five and then to three in 2003.

The loss of faith-based providers can be attributed to two factors–decreased state funding and a shift in contracting priorities. The state experienced a fiscal crisis in 2002, resulting in budget cuts in numerous programs. As the state cut budgets and as overall contracts were reduced so were faith-based dollars. In the first full year of the initiative, contracts with FBOs represented 13 percent of statewide IMPACT contracts (just over 2 million dollars). In contract year 2001-2002, these decreased to roughly 9 percent; and in 2003-2004, contracts with FBOs decreased to five percent (just over one-half million dollars). Significant cuts in the state's budget reduced both the number and size of provider contracts for both faith-based and non-faith-based organizations. In addition, the IMPACT program shifted its primary objectives away from job readiness, search, and training, toward and exclusive focus on job placement and retention. Organizations that wished to continue contracting needed to adjust their missions to fit the program's more narrow goals.

We contacted all providers in 2003. We found that 18 had an IMPACT contract at that point and 12 did not. Most of the 18 remaining IMPACT providers reported revenue stability, although the size of their IMPACT contracts had been reduced. Moreover, most NFB and MFB providers reported contracting for different services than previously. In addition, 50% of all providers reported more staff dedicated to administration and support of IMPACT and most NFB and SFB providers reported less staff involved in IMPACT service delivery. Overall, about 30% reported providing less effective services.

For the 12 providers leaving the IMPACT service delivery system, while most reported that their experience with IMPACT had been positive, their dropping out was reported as being due to decreases in IMPACT funding, their decision not to apply, or the rejection of their proposal. Being faith-based was not perceived as relevant to no longer contracting. All types of providers reported negative consequences due to the non-renewal of their contracts, including program terminations, reductions or elimination of services, and fewer staff. Most also reported that they were unable to offset the problems resulting from non-renewal.

What we experienced in Indiana may well be typical of many other local delivery systems. These types of rapid delivery system changes, however, make it more difficult to isolate the degree to which providers of various types (especially ones new to the delivery system) are performing up to expectations. By 2003, we essentially had a different delivery system, which was in many ways not comparable to what existed only a few years earlier.

CONCLUSION

In this research project, we set out with a number of goals. Over the course of the study we found answers to some of our questions, but we raised a number of others. We found, as expected, that states vary widely in their approach to the implementation of charitable choice.

This makes comparisons between states very difficult. In addition, we found out a good bit about the way faith-based providers were operating compared to their secular counterparts. The results supported some of the claims of those on both sides of the charitable choice debate. Finally, we also found some highly-tentative suggestions that client attitudes and behaviors could be influenced by FBOs.

In each case, however, our findings are limited. Upon reflection, the issues we faced are also likely to be encountered by other researchers seeking to investigate the implementation of charitable choice. For example, we only assessed one dimension of state differences, political culture, and many others could, and probably are, relevant. In terms of our provider study, it was limited to one state and considered only one service area. While differences in provider operations and outcomes could be anticipated by introducing variation on these factors, cost considerations could quickly become a serious obstacle. In addition, the entire government-funded delivery system in the two most populous areas of Indiana was composed of only 34 organizations, a number too small for the assessment of statistical significance once it is broken into the relevant subsets (FBO versus NFB, for example). Finally, we found that our delivery system was highly unstable over time.

This is not to say that research should not be done. These factors, as well as others described above, make it incumbent upon researchers to be creative and diligent in their work. In pursuing these ends, they should be able to benefit from the experiences of their colleagues. It is hoped that this paper will provide such benefits.

NOTE

1. This section relies heavily upon communication from Sheila Kennedy.

REFERENCES

Bielefeld, W. (2004). Social service delivery by faith-based organizations. *Independent Sector Memo to Members*. Washington, DC: Independent Sector.

Bielefeld, W., Littlepage, L., & Thelin, R. (2003). Results of 2001/2002 organizational nterviews. In *Faith-based social service provision under charitable choice: A study of implemenation in three states, final results* (pp. 34-49). Indianapolis, IN: Indiana University–Purdue University Indianapolis: Center for Urban Policy and the Environment.

Chambre, S. (2001). The changing nature of 'faith' in faith-based organizations: Secularization and ecumenicism in four AIDS organizations in New York City. *Social Service Review, 75,* 435-455.

Chaves, M. (2003). Debunking charitable choice: The evidence doesn't support the political left or right. *Stanford Social Innovation Review*, 1, 28-36.

Elazar, D. J. (1972). *American federalism: A view from the states* (2nd ed.). New York: Thomas Y. Crowell.

Elazar, D. J. (1984). *American federalism: A view from the states* (3rd ed.). New York: Harper & Row.

Elazar, D. J. (1986). Marketplace and commonwealth and the three political cultures. In M. Gittell (Ed.), *State politics and the new federalism* (pp. 172-179). White Plains, NY: Longman.

Elazar, D. J. (1994). The political subcultures of the United States. In *The American mosaic: The impact of space, time, and culture on American politics* (pp. 229-257). Boulder, CO: Westview Press.

Green, J. C., & Sherman A. L. (2002). *Fruitful collaborations: A survey of government-funded faith-based programs in 15 states.* Indianapolis, IN: Hudson Institute, Inc.

Jeavons, T. H. (1998). Identifying characteristics of 'religious' organizations: An exploratory proposal. In N. J. Demerath III, P. D. Hall, T. Schmitt, and R. H. Williams (Eds.), *Sacred companies: Organizational aspects of religion and religious aspects of organizations* (pp. 79-96). New York: Oxford University Press.

Jensen, L. S. (2003). Final report on the implementation of charitable choice in Massachusetts. In *Faith-based social service provision under charitable choice: A study of implemenation in three states, final results* (pp. 6-14). Indianapolis, IN: Indiana University–Purdue University Indianapolis: Center for Urban Policy and the Environment.

Johnson, B. R., Tompkins, R. B., & Webb, D. (2002*). Objective hope. Assessing the effectiveness of faith-based organizations: A review of the literature.* Philadelphia, PA: University of Pennsylvania: Center for Research on Religion and Urban Civil Society.

Littlepage, L., Thelin, R., Bielefeld, W., & Sedaca, B. (2003). Do faith-based organizations transform their clients? In *Faith-based social service provision under charitable choice: A study of implemenation in three states, final results* (62-76). Indianapolis, IN: Indiana University–Purdue University Indianapolis: Center for Urban Policy and the Environment.

McCullough, M.E., Hoyt, W.T., Larson, D.B., Koenig, H.G., & Thoresen, C. (2000). Religious involvement and mortality: A meta-analytic review. *Health Psychology*, 19, 211-222.

Mead, L.M. (2004). State political culture and welfare reform. *Policy Studies Journal*, 32, 271-296.

Monsma, S. V. (2004). *Putting faith in partnerships: Welfare-to-work in four cities.* Ann Arbor, MI: The University of Michigan Press.

Monsma, S. V., & Mounts, C. M. (2002). *Working faith: How religious organizations provide welfare-to-work services.* Philadelphia, PA: University of Pennsylvania: Center for Research on Religion and Urban Civil Society.

Search for Common Ground. (2002). *Finding common ground: 29 recommendations of the working group on human needs and faith-based and community initiatives.* Washington, DC: Search for Common Ground.

Sherman, A. L. (2003). Faith in communities: A solid investment. *Society,* January/ February, 9-26.

Smith, S. R., & Sosin, M. R. (2001). The varieties of faith-related agencies. *Public Administration Review,* 61, 651-670.

Thelin, R. (2003). Implementation of charitable choice in Indiana. In *Faith-based social service provision under charitable choice: A study of implemenation in three states, final results* (14-24). Indianpolis, IN: Indiana University–Purdue University Indianapolis: Center for Urban Policy and the Environment.

United States General Accounting Office. (2002). *Charitable choice: Overview of research findings on implementation.* Report to Congressional Requesters, GAO-02-337. Washington, DC: United States General Accounting Office.

White House, (2001). *Rallying the armies of compassion.* Retreived February 12, 2001 from *www.whitehouse.gov/news/reports/faithbased.html*

Wilson, P. (2003). Faith-based organizations, charitable choice, and government. *Administration & Society,* 35, 29-51.

Chapter 9

The Effectiveness of Faith-Based Welfare-to-Work Programs: A Story of Specialization

Stephen V. Monsma

SUMMARY. This essay first highlights three major challenges of measuring program effectiveness. It concludes effectiveness can best be conceptualized in terms of program outcomes and that such outcomes–while difficult to measure–can be measured with sufficient accuracy to justify the effort. These considerations are then illustrated by data gathered from 17 Los Angeles welfare-to-work programs and their clients in order to assess the comparative effectiveness of faith-based and secular programs. The essay concludes that no one type of welfare-to-work program was more effective across the board than any other type of program. Instead, the different types of programs seemed to be especially effective in certain specialized areas. The faith-based programs were especially effective in providing welfare recipients with emotional support and a sense of having a sympathetic, understanding base of support. The for-profit providers were especially effective in providing needed training in marketable job skills and help in finding employment. The essay

Stephen V. Monsma, PhD, is Professor Emeritus, Henry Institute for the Study of Christianity and Politics, Calvin College.

[Haworth co-indexing entry note]: "The Effectiveness of Faith-Based Welfare-to-Work Programs: A Story of Specialization." Monsma, Stephen V. Co-published simultaneously in *Journal of Religion & Spirituality in Social Work* (The Haworth Pastoral Press, an imprint of The Haworth Press, Inc.) Vol. 25, No. 3/4, 2006, pp. 175-195; and: *Faith-Based Social Services: Measures, Assessments, and Effectiveness* (ed: Stephanie C. Boddie, and Ram A. Cnaan) The Haworth Pastoral Press, an imprint of The Haworth Press, Inc., 2006, pp. 175-195.

concludes by discussing two public policy implications that flow from this type of program specialization.

KEYWORDS. Program effectiveness, welfare programs, faith-based programs

The assertion that the systematic study of the effectiveness of faith-based social service programs is extremely difficult has risen–or sunk–to the level of a truism. As many have pointed out, the challenges are many and the existing studies that point the way are few (Miller, 1999; Sowa, Selden, and Sandfort, 2004; and Flynn and Hodgkinson, 2001). In fact, not only are there very few systematic studies of the effectiveness of faith-based social service programs, there are very few systematic studies of the effectiveness of social service programs of any type. Even more rare, and more challenging, are studies that compare the effectiveness of different types of social service programs.

In this essay I seek, first, briefly to present three difficulties in comparative effectiveness research that I have found especially challenging. Next, I present some of my research findings on the comparative effectiveness of different types of welfare-to-work programs, in an attempt both to illustrate these three difficulties and to demonstrate how they can be at least partially overcome. In the final section, I suggest two policy conclusions that can be drawn from the research findings I present. I believe effectiveness research can be done and–even with the challenges it presents–can yield useful insights and point the way to more effective public policies.

THREE CHALLENGING DIFFICULTIES

The first challenge a researcher studying the effectiveness of social service programs confronts is that of defining effectiveness. Different researchers have defined it differently. Some have defined effectiveness in terms of certain organizational factors that the researchers perceive as being important. They have focused on such measures of organizational health as an active, involved board of directors, low staff turnover, and adequate funding for the programs that have been undertaken. Another approach to defining effectiveness focuses on certain factors or forces external to an organization and assesses the success or failure of the organization in dealing with those factors. Examples of such external factors include funding and referral agencies, key community leaders, and political actors or processes crucial to the organization's health. This approach focuses on the organization's acquisition of resources and its relationship with external actors that are important to its ability to function successfully.

Other effectiveness studies have defined effectiveness in terms of the products being produced by the social service programs under study: the number of clients assisted, the number of meals served, the hours of counseling sessions provided, the hours of classroom instruction given, and so forth. Sometimes a further step is taken and the cost of each such unit of service is calculated. This enables one to compare the cost per unit of service being offered by different providers. One can also define effectiveness in terms of client evaluations of the programs they have been in. Both a respect for the worth and dignity of program clients and a belief that those who are recipients of services are in the best position to judge its effectiveness argue in favor of this approach to defining effectiveness. Private, for-profit businesses often use "customer satisfaction" as a gauge of how well they are doing; the effectiveness of social service programs can be similarly defined.

All four of these concepts of effectiveness, however, suffer from a failure to consider the extent to which the social service programs under study actually achieve their intended results or goals. While information on organizational health, or on its relationship to its key environmental forces, or on the number and costs of the products or outputs of a social service program, or on client evaluations are helpful, what they ignore are the results or outcomes of the provision of an agency's services. Whether or not persons are becoming drug-free, or are finding jobs, or are passing the GRE, or are learning English–or whatever else the goal of the program may be–is left unknown. A program could have a great management structure in place, have a well-educated, stable, and highly satisfied work force, be producing the services it was designed to produced in a cost effective manner, have highly positive relationships with key actors in its environment, and receive highly positive evaluations from the persons it is serving, but still post very dismal results in terms of the final purposes for which it was created. The possible examples are many: a well run high school with a high dropout rate and students who are not learning, an ex-offender reentry program with low costs per ex-offender served but very high recidivism rates, and a welfare-to-work program that is widely respected by key actors in the community but with few persons finding employment. It is reasonable to assume that such programs will be the exception–one would presume that positive program characteristics will usually be related to positive program results–but there is no guarantee this will always be the case. As I will argue shortly, client evaluations are especially likely to be closely related to program outcomes, and surely highly negative client evaluations are likely to presage a lack of positive outcomes. But even they do not focus directly on program outcomes.

Thus, many have argued that the preferred definition of program effectiveness focuses on program outcomes, that is, on the results or consequences of the services being provided. It centers in on the question of the extent to which the goals or purposes of the program are being achieved. This definition of effectiveness has the big advantage of spotlighting the success or failure of an organization in achieving that which it was established to achieve. Especially from a public policy point of view–where the emphasis is on the positive results for clients and ultimately for society as a whole that are or are not being attained–defining effectiveness in terms of outcomes actually achieved has many advantages.

President Bush's faith-based and community initiative–which has sought to enable more faith-based and small, community-based social service programs to compete successfully for government funding–has led more policy makers and policy analysts to ask the question of whether or not faith-based and community-based social service programs are more successful than their secular and larger, more professionalized counterparts. Some advocates of Bush's faith-based and community initiative have claimed faith-based agencies have achieved spectacular results (Towey, 2002). Others have pointed out there are few, if any, empirically rigorous studies demonstrating more positive outcomes for clients of faith-based programs (Gill, 2004). The issue here is clearly that of program effectiveness conceptualized in terms of program outcomes or results.

If one defines effectiveness in terms of program outcomes, it is helpful to distinguish between what can be termed enabling, intermediate, and ultimate outcomes. Ultimate outcomes focus on the end-product or final result the program is designed to achieve: drug-free persons for a drug rehabilitation program, persons with self-supporting employment for a welfare-to-work program, or persons avoiding arrest and conviction for an ex-offenders' re-entry program. There are also intermediate outcomes. These are outcomes which, while less than the desired ultimate outcome, are markers of notable progress towards achieving an ultimate outcome. For an ex-offenders program these might include finding gainful employment, or meeting the conditions of one's probation. For a drug rehabilitation program intermediate outcomes might include successfully completing a drug withdrawal program, or staying off drugs for a set, but limited amount of time. There are also enabling outcomes. These are outcomes that, while not marking the achievement of the program's ultimate goal or even marking the partial achievement of or movement towards an ultimate outcome, will likely work to make achievement of ultimate or intermediate outcomes more likely. For a welfare recipient who does not know English, completing an ESL (English as a second language) course of study would be an example of an enabling outcome for a welfare-to-work program. It is not the ultimate outcome of finding self-supporting employment, nor even an intermediate outcome, such as finding part-time employment or employment at less than a self-supporting level. Yet it is an outcome that will enable, or make more likely, the client achieving intermediate and ultimate outcomes. Positive evaluations of a program by its clients should also be considered an enabling outcome. They indicate a program was successful in connecting with its clients in a positive, constructive manner, presumably a minimum–or enabling–condition for achieving positive ultimate and intermediate outcomes.

However, even if researchers define effectiveness in terms of outcomes, their challenges are not over. I have experienced two additional, hard-to-solve-problems, when seeking to compare the outcome effectiveness of two different programs or two different types of programs. Yet for policy makers deciding whether public policy ought to favor one or the other type of program and for public or private decision-makers choosing to award a grant or contract to one social service provider or another, this is often the most crucial question to answer. It lies at the heart of the dispute over the relative effectiveness of faith-based and community-based social service providers, compared to large, professionalized, secular providers.

The first one of these two additional problems is how to measure accurately the outcomes of difference programs or program types. Especially difficult is the challenge of controlling for the fact that the programs one is seeking to compare may have different types of clients to begin with. If faith-based programs, for example, tend to have clients who are facing more difficult barriers to their achieving success than the clients of similar secular programs, it would be no wonder if they did not have as positive outcomes as do the secular programs. One potential way to overcome this challenge is to assign clients randomly to the various programs. In this way one could be assured that no program or type of program is starting out with a predominance of clients either especially easy or especially challenging with whom to work. There are, however, both practical and theoretical problems in using random assignment as a means to control for different programs having different types of client with whom to work. Practically, it is usually impossible to engage in random assignment of clients to different program types if faith-based programs are involved, since persons under charitable choice and presumably under the First Amendment may not be required to take part in a faith-based program if they would prefer a secular alternative. There is the added practical problem that, even if random assignment could be followed, the clients would soon figure out what sort of a program they are in, and this knowledge could affect the outcomes. Government and for-profit programs, for example, might carry a negative stigma in some persons' minds and that in itself might reduce the chances of those persons experiencing positive outcomes. One is facing a much more difficult situation than does a drug company doing a double blind study in order to test the effectiveness of a new drug.

There are also theoretical problems in the random assignment model. It has a hidden assumption; namely, that different types of programs are or should be equally effective with all types of persons. It is a one-size-fits-all assumption. This needs to be challenged. For example, in terms of assignment to a faith-based versus a secular program, think of two persons, one for whom religion has played an important part in her life since childhood. She is still actively involved in a church and thinks of herself as a child of a loving God. Another person is very antagonistic to religion. He has bad memories of a harsh, condemning religion while growing up, has no use for religion in any form, and has sworn never to darken the doors of a church again. It takes no great insight to realize that a deeply faith-oriented drug treatment program, for example, is much more likely to achieve positive results with the first person than the second, and that a thoroughly secular program is more likely to achieve positive results with the second person than the first. To take another example, randomly assigning Latino clients to two different social service programs, one of which is staffed predominantly by Latinos and one of which is staffed predominantly by "Anglos," assumes that the ethnic or racial make up a program's staff is irrelevant. This flies in the face of common sense.

Researchers can attempt to control by statistical means, such as regression analysis, the effect of background characteristics of the clients of the different program types. This is usually the best answer to this challenge to the researcher. But to do this researchers must decide which background characteristics are likely to prove important and therefore worth gathering data on. In the process, they may miss some characteristics that in fact it would have been important to include. This can especially be the case in regard to more nebulous, hard-to-discern characteristics of attitude and motivation. Also, one needs very large numbers of participants in one's study in order to come up with statistically significant results. Confidentiality issues may also arise as one probes into the background of the different programs' clients.

And this is not the end of the challenges researchers face in accurately measuring program outcomes. There is the issue of clients who have dropped out of a program before completing it. Ought they, and their successes or failures, to be included in a study of program outcomes? One can, of course, question whether it is fair to judge a program by persons who began it but did not complete it. After all they did not have the full benefit of the program. In fact, some might drop out after only taking part very briefly in it. In such cases to judge a program on the basis of individuals who barely took part in it seems unfair. But if a program has a high drop-out rate, it also seems unfair to only judge it by those who stick it out to the end. Intent-to-treat analysis argues it is important to consider the results experienced by all persons who begin a program and not only by those who complete it. Otherwise one is considering the outcomes of the program for persons who are less than representative of the entire client population (Houck, Mazumdar, Liu, and Reynolds, 2000). Outcome research is indeed not easy!

A final challenge in comparative outcome research lies in the fact that social service providers often differ in multiple ways. Thus, if their outcomes differ, what of the many attributes by which they differ ought one to credit the differing outcomes? For example, the question is often asked if faith-based programs experience better outcomes than do their secular counterparts. But faith-based and secular social service programs may differ in more ways than in the presence or absence of a religious dimension. Faith-based agencies may be much smaller, more community-based, and less professionalized. They may pursue different methodologies or approaches to achieving the desired goals. Thus, if faith-based programs are found to be more, or less, effective than secu-

lar programs in terms of client outcomes, how does one tell if the observed differences are due to the presence or absence of the faith element or due to other differences, such as size, community orientation,
level of professionalization, or methodologies utilized?

In short, when it comes to effectiveness research the challenges and
pitfalls lurk everywhere. But this is different than saying that meaningful effectiveness research cannot be done. I believe it can. It is difficult
and one ought to proceed with caution and ought not to claim more than
one should for one's findings. But I am convinced meaningful effectiveness research can be done, research that can be of help to policy
makers in and out of government. In the following sections of this essay
I illustrate both the possibilities and the challenges one faces in studying
the effectiveness of faith-based social service programs compared to
that of their secular counterparts, by presenting some findings from a
study of welfare-to-work programs in which I have been engaged. I will
illustrate how I dealt with three of the key challenges outlined above–
controlling for program differences other than the faith element, controlling for program dropouts, and controlling for differing background
characteristics of program clients–and how my findings can be used to
inform public policies.

PROGRAM DIFFERENCES
OTHER THAN THE FAITH ELEMENT

In this section I first illustrate that faith-based and secular welfare-to-work programs in fact differ in more ways than the faith element, and then show how that fact can be taken into account in analyzing
and presenting one's data. In this section and in the following two sections I will be drawing on data a colleague of mine and I gathered in a
study of 17 welfare-to-work programs in Los Angeles. Thus, I first need
to briefly introduce this study and how we went about conducting it
(Monsma and Soper, 2003 and Monsma and Soper, forthcoming).[1] By
way of a mailed questionnaire we gathered information 200 welfare-
to-work programs in Los Angeles County which by several measures
were representative of all such programs in Los Angeles County, we
next divided them into government, for-profit, secular nonprofit, and
faith-based programs, and then selected 17 programs from the four
types of programs that possessed characteristics typical of their program types. We selected 3 government-run programs, 2 for-profit programs, 4 secular nonprofit programs, and 8 faith-based programs. We

obtained additional information on these programs by way of site visits. We also obtained baseline data from clients of these programs who were participating in the programs at the time of our study. By way of telephone interviews six months and then twelve months later we obtained information on the clients' evaluations of the programs that had been in, program completion rates, and current employment status.

First, this study was able to confirm that the faith-based programs and the government and for-profit programs go about welfare-to-work in somewhat different ways, apart from the presence or absence of a religious dimension. Researchers and practitioners in the welfare-to-work area often make a distinction between soft skills training and hard skills training (Moss and Tilly, 2001:44). Soft skills consist of attitudes, values, and forms of behavior that are conducive to obtaining, holding, and advancing in a job. Examples include training in appropriate workplace dress, punctuality, setting career goals, self-esteem, the importance and value of work, and anger management. Hard skills consist of vocational and job skills, as well as basic skills, such as reading and computational skills, that make employment more likely. From an earlier study of mine of welfare-to-work programs in Los Angeles, Dallas, Chicago, and Philadelphia it is clear that faith-based programs tend to put a greater relative emphasis on soft skills training and the large government and for-profit programs on hard skills training (Monsma, 2004:102-105). Among the faith-based programs about 38 percent of all of the services they offered involved soft skills, while in the government programs only about 25 percent of their services were in soft skills and 31 percent of the for-profit programs' services were in soft skills. Even more illuminating is the more detailed study of the 17 Los Angeles welfare-to-work programs my colleague and I conducted. Based on site visits and interviews with staff, we found that five of the eight faith-based programs we studied emphasized training in soft skills to the near exclusion of hard skills training. With only one exception the six government and for-profit programs clearly emphasized vocational training and the development of hard, marketable skills. This pattern was confirmed by the six-month telephone interviews with 327 clients of the 17 programs. We asked them two open-ended questions about what in their welfare-to-work programs was most helpful to them and if they had any comments, ideas, or suggestions in regard to the program they had been in. We found that of the 86 comments made in response to these two open-ended questions by faith-based program respondents, 26 percent mentioned training or help in skills that would be classified as soft skills, while only 12 percent mentioned training in hard skills. In contrast, of the 186 comments made by respondents who had attended a government or a for-profit program only 9 percent mentioned training in soft skills and 47 percent mentioned training in hard skills.

Other studies have come up with similar findings. A team of researchers, for example, studied welfare-to-work providers in three counties in Indiana (Bielefeld, Littlepage, and Thelin, 2003). They categorized the programs as being ones with no faith influence, a moderate level of faith influence, and a strong level of faith influence. They report they found that all three types of programs provided about the same number of soft skills services, but that the no-faith-influence and moderate-faith-influence programs were providing about twice the number of hard skills services than were the strong-faith-influence programs. In other words, the strong-faith-influenced programs were putting a greater relative emphasis on soft skills training. Other studies have produced similar results (Goggin and Orth, 2002, and Lockhart, 2001).

Thus one immediately faces the problem in evaluating faith-based welfare-to-work program outcomes of determining whether any observed differences are due to the soft skills emphasis of the faith-based programs or due to their religious nature or emphasis. In this section of my essay I use client evaluations as an effectiveness measure. Although client evaluations are neither the ultimate outcome of a welfare-to-work program nor even an intermediate outcome, as seen earlier they can be considered an enabling outcome.

In an attempt to disentangle the soft versus hard skills training from the faith-based versus government or for-profit character of the programs, I first divided the eight faith-based programs into the five that emphasized soft skills training and the three that emphasized hard skills training, and I also divided the six government and for-profit programs into the five that emphasized hard skills training and the one government program that emphasized soft skills training. I thereby ended up with four program types: faith-based with a soft skills emphasis, faith-based with a hard skills emphasis, government and for-profit with a soft skills emphasis, and government and for-profit with a soft skills emphasis. I did not include the clients from three secular nonprofit programs in this analysis since by several measures they combined characteristics of the faith-based and of the government and for-profit programs and I wanted to focus here on the sharply contrasting programs.

In the six-month telephone interviews with these programs' clients the respondents were asked to assess their programs' staff and overall helpfulness to them by way of five evaluative questions. Table 1 gives four of these evaluative questions and the respondents' answers to them

TABLE 1. Client Evaluations of Programs

Statement asked of respondents:	Always true	Sometimes true	Never true	Total	
				N	%
The people running or teaching in [name of program] were people who took an interest in me personally.					
Faith-based programs, soft skills emphasis	60%	34%	6%	47	100%
Faith-based programs, hard skills emphasis	80%	20%	0%	25	100%
Govt. program, soft skills emphasis	54%	39%	8%	13	101%
Govt. for-profit programs, hard skills emphasis	49%	45%	5%	152	99%
The people running or teaching [name of program] were people who really cared about my problems.					
Faith-based programs, soft skills emphasis	66%	21%	13%	47	100%
Faith-based programs, hard skills emphasis	65%	26%	9%	23	100%
Govt. program, soft skills emphasis	62%	31%	8%	13	101%
Govt. for-profit programs, hard skills emphasis	46%	38%	16%	151	100%
The people running or teaching [name of program] were people who understood me and the situation I was in.					
Faith-based programs, soft skills emphasis	68%	19%	13%	47	100%
Faith-based programs, hard skills emphasis	65%	26%	9%	23	100%
Govt. program, soft skills emphasis	54%	31%	15%	13	100%
Govt. for-profit programs, hard skills emphasis	50%	40%	10%	152	100%
The people running or teaching [name of program] were people who were knowledgeable about how to help me.					
Faith-based programs, soft skills emphasis	60%	31%	8%	48	99%
Faith-based programs, hard skills emphasis	68%	32%	0%	23	100%
Govt. program, soft skills emphasis	69%	23%	8%	13	100%
Govt. for-profit programs, hard skills emphasis	65%	27%	8%	152	100%

(the responses to the fifth one are included in Table 2). On the first three questions the faith-based programs tended to be evaluated more positively than did the secular government and for-profit programs, whether they emphasized soft or hard skills training. These three questions inquired concerning the programs' staffs' levels of personal interest, concern, and understanding. About two-thirds of the faith-based clients

TABLE 2. Client Evaluations of Helpfulness of Their Programs

Question asked of respondents:	Very helpful	Some-what helpful	Not helpful at all	Total	
				N	%
Was [name of program] very helpful to you, somewhat helpful to you, or not at all helpful to you?					
Faith-based programs, soft skills emphasis	58%	25%	17%	48	100%
Faith-based programs, hard skills emphasis	63%	33%	4%	24	100%
Govt. program, soft skills emphasis	62%	23%	15%	13	100%
Govt. for-profit programs, hard skills emphasis	67%	28%	5%	150	100%

indicated that it was "always true" that their program staffs possessed these personal qualities of interest, concern, and understanding, while about one-half of the government and for-profit clients did so. Although, the differences were small, on all three questions the clients of the government program that emphasized soft skills training rated their program's staff slightly more positively than did the secular programs that emphasized hard skills training.

These findings suggest that although a soft-skills emphasis by a welfare-to-work program may increase the positive client evaluations of the level of concern and understanding of a program's staff, the faith-based character of the program does so to an even greater degree. The religious or nonreligious nature of the programs seems to be more important than the soft skills versus hard skills emphasis of the program.

The fourth question included in Table 1 and the question included in Table 2, however, tell a slightly different story. The fourth question in Table 1 inquired concerning the clients' perception of the level of knowledgeableness of their programs' staffs and Table 2 gives the results of a question that asked about the overall helpfulness of the programs. These two questions thereby focused on the practical, helpful qualities of the programs and their staffs, while the three earlier questions dealt with the supportive, empathic nature of the programs' staffs. The question about the staffs' knowledgeableness elicited about the same level of positive responses, whether the programs were faith-based or secular and soft-skills or hard-skills oriented. Table 2 reveals that a majority of the clients of all four program types rated their programs as being "very helpful," but larger majorities of clients in the hard skills programs did so than did the soft skills program clients. Also, fifteen percent of the soft skills government program clients said it was of no help at all, and 17 percent of the soft skills faith-based programs said the same thing–both notably higher than their hard-skills-emphasis counterparts.

From this one can reach two conclusions. First, the clients of faith-based, soft-skill training programs were reacting to their soft-skills training in a highly positive manner. They felt that the instructors or counselors they had had in these programs were understanding and supportive and that they knew how to help them. Overall, they felt their programs had been helpful to them. Clearly, they thought the soft-skills training they had received, given in a religious context, had been a positive experience and helpful to them. Second, the clients of the secular programs, while evaluating their program staff less positively in terms of thoughtfulness and concern, evaluated their programs more positively in terms of overall helpfulness, *but only if those programs also had a hard skills emphasis.*

These findings illustrate the possibilities of using the evaluations of the participants in a program as a measure of program effectiveness conceptualized as an enabling outcome, and also both the importance and possibilities of taking into account not only the faith-based or secular nature of programs, but also other ways in which faith-based and secular programs may differ.

PROGRAM COMPLETION

Completion of a welfare-to-work program can also be considered an enabling outcome. For persons struggling to survive on welfare completing a program in itself is a major achievement. Doing so is evidence of a participant's ability to set a goal and then to persist in achieving it. This involves many of the same skills or resources one needs to succeed in the work place: solving childcare and transportation challenges, learning to keep a schedule, and persevering in a commitment once made. Many welfare-to-work programs I visited had elaborate "graduation" ceremonies to mark the end of a program, with members of clients' families in attendance and recognition and praise heaped on those who had completed the program. Thus, the simple fact of completing a program may appropriately be considered an enabling outcome; it certainly is evidence of the presence of key attitudes and skills that are enabling outcomes. It should be kept in mind that the 17 programs included in this study varied in length and intensity. Thus completing some programs involved more effort than did completing others of the programs. Nevertheless, I felt that success in taking on and achieving a goal–whether major or modest–constitutes a significant enabling outcome. For this analysis I separated four faith-based programs that made certain religious elements explicit and integrated them into their programming (faith-based/integrated) from four whose religious elements were largely implicit and separate from their programming (faith-based/segmented).

Table 3 shows that by this measure the for-profit and faith-based/integrated programs were the most effective, with only 8 and 14 percent of their clients dropping out before completing their programs, although the government programs were not far behind, with a 19 percent failure-to-complete rate. The nonprofit/secular and faith-based/segmented clients fared the worst, with about 40 percent of them not completing their programs. I will comment on the for-profit programs' success in the next section of this essay, when I consider employment outcomes. It is difficult to explain the much higher completion rate for respondents in the integrally religious faith-based programs as compared to those in the faith-based groups that did not explicitly integrate religious elements into their programming. Since all three of the faith-based groups that emphasized hard skills rather than soft skills were faith-based/segmented programs, one might supposed that this might explain the difference. But it does not. There were no differences between the one faith-based/segmented programs that emphasized soft skills training and the three that emphasized hard skills training. Nor did the two types of

TABLE 3. Percent of Respondents Who Failed to Complete Their Programs

Program type:	Percent who did not complete program[a]	N
Government	19%	96
For-profit	8%	91
Nonprofit/secular	40%	66
Faith-based/segmented	39%	36
Faith-based/integrated	14%	36

[a]That is, the percent of clients who at the baseline were in a welfare-to-work program, but at six months reported that for some reason had not completed it, but left early. The vast majority of those who did not fall into this category had successfully completed the program, although a few were still in the program at six months.

faith-based programs differ in their clients evaluations of their staffs' supportiveness or helpfulness (the questions on which the prior section reported). One is led to conclude that the explicit religious content itself of the faith-based/integrated programs may have encouraged program completion. But this conclusion can also be questioned since the for-profit programs, which had no religious content, had an even slightly higher completion rate than the faith-based/integrated programs. It may be that either an explicit religious element or the qualities of the for-profit programs to be discussed shortly led to high completion rates.

EMPLOYMENT OUTCOMES

The key positive outcome for welfare-to-work programs is their success in enabling their clients to secure employment, especially full-time employment. Even though securing full-time employment is no guarantee of totally escaping the need for welfare assistance, the absence of full-time employment is almost a certain guarantee of needing continued welfare assistance. Full-time employment is a crucial intermediate outcome and comes close to being the ultimate outcome of welfare-to-work programs.

In order to solve the challenge of different results for different types of programs perhaps being caused simply by certain programs having clients with characteristics that make it easier or harder for them to find employment and leave welfare, I used logistic regression analysis to assess which variables were statistically significant in predicting the full-time employment of respondents at six and twelve months. This is a statistical technique that measures the independent impact that each of a number of variables has on the outcome one is seeking to explain. In this case here I was seeking to explain the full-time employment status of the respondents. As discussed earlier, this status could be affected not only by the type of program in which they had taken part, but also by such factors as race, number of dependent children, gender, education level, and so forth. Logistic regression analysis enables one to answer the question of what impact each of these factors, or variables, had on the employment status of the respondents, if all of the other variables are held constant. Thus, for example, it answers the question of what was the independent impact on employment of having taken part in a faith-based welfare-to-work program if other variables, such as education, race, and gender are the same.

The results of this analysis are reported in Table 4. I considered 30 hours or more of work a week as full-time employment. At six months there were four statistically significant relationships. Being female and being unemployed at the baseline, significantly decreased one's chances of finding full-time employment, and being unmarried significantly increased the chances of one doing so. Most interestingly for my purposes here, being in a for-profit program significantly increased one's chances of finding full-time employment (as compared to being in a government

TABLE 4. Determinants of Full-Time Employment at 6 and 12 Months

Predictor Variable:	Full-Time Employment at 6 Months	Full-Time Employment at 12 Months
Gender		
Female	−.95**	−.40
Male (reference category)	—	—
Race		
Black	−.55	−.48
Latino	.10	.30
Other Race	−.28	−.08
White (reference category)	—	—
Employment Status		
Unemployed	−.67**	−.38
Employed (reference category)	—	—
Number of Work-Related Skills[a]	.16	.04
Marital Status		
Unmarried	.89**	1.00**
Married (reference category)	—	—
Number of Children	.03	.12
Type of Welfare-to-Work-Program		
For-profit	1.13**	1.14**
Nonprofit/secular	.03	.23
Faith-based/segmented	.56	.66
Faith-based/integrated	.58	.12
Government (reference category)	—	—
N	327	265
Nagelkirche R Square	.16	.15

*$p < .10$. ** $p < .05$.
[a] Number of work-related skills is a scale of 0-3 based on the sum of having a high school education, being able to read English, and being able to speak English.
Note. Numbers from each column are the logistic regression coefficients.

program), even when all the other variables listed in Table 4 are held constant. Both types of faith-based programs had positive coefficient scores when compared to the government programs, but they were too small to say with confidence whether or not these scores resulted merely by chance. One cannot say with confidence their clients were doing better at full-time employment than were the government programs. The same can be said for the nonprofit/secular programs, although their coefficient scores were even lower than those of the faith-based programs. Here the importance of having larger numbers of respondents than what I had in this study is seen. Achieving statistical significance is a function of both the observed patterns and the number of respondents included in one's study. Even when the observed patterns do not change, they are less and less likely to be have been caused by chance as the numbers of respondents included in the study increase.

Table 4 shows there were some changes at twelve months. Being female or unemployed at the baseline no longer decreased one's chances of finding employment, while being unmarried continued to increase one's chances of finding a job. Meanwhile, being in a for-profit program continued to significantly increase one's chances of finding full-time employment, as it did at six months. Both types of faith-based programs continued to have positive coefficient scores; both continued to fail to reach statistical significance.

These findings demonstrate the effectiveness of the for-profit programs in enabling their clients to find full-time employment. At both the six month and twelve month interviews, even when one holds constant gender, race, baseline employment status, work-related skills (including education), marital status, and the number of dependent children, the for-profit program clients did significantly better than the government program clients in finding full-time employment. This was true of no other type of program, including the faith-based programs.

From my knowledge of these 17 programs three possible reasons suggest themselves for this for-profit program success. One is the focused, job-training emphasis of the for-profit programs included in this study. The for-profit programs were vocational education programs, and although they had some supportive services in addition to the job skills classes, the emphasis was clearly on the skills training. Also, both had internship programs, which in themselves may have been a factor in their clients' success in finding full-time employment. Second, the for-profit programs clearly felt themselves under the gun and in need of producing positive results. The use of for-profit firms to provide welfare-to-work services in Los Angeles County had been highly controversial and accompanied by high-profile newspaper stories (Riccardi, June 21, 2000:4, July 12, 2000:B3). As a result the for-profit programs felt they were under scrutiny and were experiencing strong pressures to produce positive results. That was a part of their culture. A third possible explanation for the high levels of employment success of the for-profit providers is that the variables I included in my regression analysis may have missed some important client characteristics that marked the for-profit clients and predisposed them to success. I took all of the obvious–and some not-so-obvious–variables into account, but there may be others that I missed. In particular, certain habits of mind or motivation that could not be included in the variables I selected for analysis may have played a part. This possibility illustrates a challenge that is not totally removed, even when sophisticated statistical techniques such as logistic regression analysis is used. That is why studies that replicate this study are important. It is only as additional studies are done in different cities and different settings that what I found here in this study will be reaffirmed or shown to be in need of modification. These three factors may also help explain the previously-discussed high program completion rates of the for-profit providers' clients.

Lastly, a finding helpful to note is that those respondents who attended a faith-based program and reported they already had a job at the time of the baseline did better at maintaining employment than did those respondents who already had a job and attended other types of programs. (The jobs that some of the respondents had at the time of the baseline survey were generally part-tine jobs.) At six months about 90 percent had done so and at twelve over 80 percent had done so. The respondents from the other program types fell into the 60 or 70 percent range. This finding may relate to the earlier finding that the faith-based clients found their programs to be highly supportive and understanding of them. If a person already had a job, the highly supportive, soft skills emphasis of a faith-based program may have enabled them to maintain employment, while the less supportive, hard skills emphasis of the other program types may have resulted in their clients with jobs not experiencing the supportive environment helpful in keeping them. Since many in the field have held that maintaining employment is a greater challenge for welfare-dependent persons than finding an initial job, this aspect of faith-based program effectiveness is worth noting.

SUMMARY AND POLICY CONCLUSIONS

The findings I have reported here indicate that it is much too easy to conclude that welfare-to-work programs of any one type were generally more effective than other types of programs. Instead, my findings tell a story of specialization: some types of programs were good at achieving certain types of outcomes; other types of programs were good at achieving other types of outcomes. The faith-based programs were especially effective in three ways: in creating a sympathetic, supportive atmosphere for their clients, in enabling their clients to complete the welfare-to-work programs once they had begun them (for the faith-based/integrated programs only), and in enabling their clients who were already employed to maintain their employment. Meanwhile, the for-profit programs were especially effective in the crucial outcome of enabling their clients to obtain full-time employment. The program types were evaluated by their clients as being about equally effective in terms of their practical helpfulness.

These findings are more tentative than definitive. Further research may demonstrate they are need of modification–or even complete reversal. As I argued early in this essay, effectiveness research is not easy. But I am convinced these findings are empirically defensible, give us new insights into the nature of faith-based social service organizations, and carry with them a number of helpful public policy implications.

More specifically, I would suggest these findings suggest two conclusions highly relevant to welfare-to-work public policy. First, they suggest there is no reason either to exclude faith-based providers from government contracts for welfare-to-work services or to embrace massive shifts of government resources to faith-based welfare-to-work providers. Neither faith-based providers nor their secular counterparts proved to be more effective across the board. The faith-based providers were more effective by some outcome measures and no more or even less successful by other outcome measures. To me, this suggests faith-based providers should be included in the mix of providers with whom government forms financial partnerships, but that primary reliance on them is not warranted.

Second, my findings lend support for what William Galston has termed niche effectiveness, that is, the position that different types of social service providers may have their own specialized niches in which they excel. He has suggested that perhaps there is "such a niche or niches in the general area of social welfare and social service provision such that religious congregations and faith-based organizations are uniquely well suited to fill that niche or niches" (Galston, 2003:2). The research reported here suggests that the specialized niche in which faith-based organizations excel is that of providing welfare recipients with the emotional support and a sense of having a sympathetic, understanding base of support. These sorts of supports may enable persons on welfare to persevere in completing a training program and in overcoming attitudinal and practical obstacles to maintaining employment once a job has been found. Meanwhile, the specialization in which for-profit providers may excel is in providing needed training in marketable job skills and help in finding employment. The most effective welfare-to-work approach may be one that makes use of both of these specialized strengths, using faith-based programs to provide soft-skills training and the supportive sense of empathy many persons need in a highly competitive job market, and using the for-profit programs to provide the job skills training many persons also need.

Whether or not subsequent effectiveness research or possible pilot programs prove these policy suggestions to be accurate or mistaken is less important than the fact that even with all the challenges that effectiveness researchers face, useful research on the comparative effectiveness of different types of providers can be done. This research can offer guidance to policy makers. The established facts on welfare-to-work program successes and failures and the guidance these facts can give policy makers are less certain and thinner than what one would want in an ideal world. Nevertheless, policy decisions are made every day on fewer facts and with less guidance than is available from findings such as the ones I have described in this essay. Comparative effectiveness research–even with all the challenges it faces–is worth doing and can yield useful information with practical applications.

NOTE

1. This research was supported by a grant from the John and Dora Randolph Haynes Foundation of Los Angeles, with some supplemental funding from the Smith-Richardson Foundation and Pepperdine University.

REFERENCES

Bielefeld, Wolfgang, Laura Littlepage, and Rachel Thelin (2003). Organizational Analysis: The Influence of Faith on IMPACT Service Providers. In *Charitable Choice: First Results from Three States,* edited by Sheila Suess Kennedy and Wolfgang Bielefeld, pp. 57-64. Indianapolis, IN: Center for Urban Policy and the

Environment, School of Public and Environmental Affairs, Indiana University-Purdue University, Indianapolis.

Flynn, Patrice and Virginia A. Hodgkinson (Eds.), (2001). *Measuring the Impact of the Nonprofit Sector.* New York: Kluwer Academic/Plenum.

Galston, William. (2003). Breakout Session: Faith-Based Service Niches. The Roundtable of Religion and Social Welfare Policy, Spring Research Forum.

Gill, Emily R. (2004). Religious Organizations, Charitable Choice, and the Limits of Freedom of Conscience. *Perspectives on Politics,* 2(4): 741-755.

Goggin, Malcolm L. and Deborah A. Orth. (2002). How Faith-Based and Secular Organizations Tackle Housing for the Homeless. A report presented at the Roundtable on Religion and Social Welfare Policy, Rockefeller Institute of Government.

Houck, Patricia R., Sati Mazumdar, Kenneth S Liu, and Charles F. Reynolds III. (2000). A Pragmatic Intent-to-Treat Analysis Using SAS. A paper presented at the Northeast SAS Users Group conference, Philadelphia, PA. Available at: http://www.nesug.org/html/Proceedings/nesug00/st/st9008.pdf

Lockhart, William, H. (2001). Getting Saved from Poverty: Religion in Poverty-to-Work Programs. PhD dissertation, Department of Sociology, University of Virginia.

Miller, D. W. (November 26, 1999). Measuring the Role of the "Faith Factor" in Social Change. *Chronicle of Higher Education*: A21.

Monsma, Stephen V. (2004). *Putting Faith in Partnerships: Welfare-to-Work in Four Cities.* Ann Arbor, MI: University of Michigan Press.

_____ and J. Christopher Soper. (Forthcoming). *Enabling Those in Need: Comparing the Outcomes of Welfare-to-Work Programs in Los Angeles.* Washington, DC: Georgetown University Press.

_____. (2003). *What Works: Comparing the Effectiveness of Welfare-to-Work Programs in Los Angeles.* Philadelphia, PA: Center for Research on Religion and Urban Civil Society, University of Pennsylvania.

Moss, Philip and Chris Tilly. (2001). *Stories Employers Tell: Race, Skill, and Hiring in America.* New York: Russell Sage Foundation.

Riccardi, Nicholas. (June 21, 2000). Political Struggle Centers on Welfare-to-Work Contractor. *Los Angeles Times*: B4.

_____. (July 12, 2000). Supervisors Privatize Job-Training Services. *Los Angeles Times:* B3.

Sowa, Jessica E., Sally Coleman Selden, and Jodi R. Sandfort. (2004). No Longer Unmeasurable? A Multidimensional Integrated Model of Nonprofit Organizational Effectiveness. *Nonprofit and Voluntary Sector Quarterly* 33(4): 711-728.

Towey, Jim. (2002). Next Steps for the President's Faith-Based Initiative. Speech given as a part of the Heritage Foundation Lectures, No. 752.

Chapter 10

A Faith-Based Alternative Youth Education Program: Evaluating a Participatory Research Approach

Jill Witmer Sinha

SUMMARY. Community-based and faith-based programs are on-going partners in the social welfare mix which characterizes U.S. welfare provision. In the face of calls for more rigorous research on the capacity and impact of faith-based and community-based programs which use public funds, the research community must gain sophistication in addressing methodological issues inherent in participatory designs for the study of such programs. This article describes concerns which arose while implementing participatory research during a federally-funded, intensive 10-month long case study of a faith-based alternative education program for at risk youth. The project was funded through the Department of Health and Humans Services, Administration for Children

Jill Witmer Sinha, PhD, is affiliated with Princeton University, Center for Study of Religion.

Address correspondence to: Jill Witmer Sinha, 5 Ivy Lane, Princeton, NJ 08544 (E-mail: jsinha@princeton.edu).

[Haworth co-indexing entry note]: "A Faith-Based Alternative Youth Education Program: Evaluating a Participatory Research Approach." Sinha, Jill Witmer. Co-published simultaneously in *Journal of Religion & Spirituality in Social Work* (The Haworth Pastoral Press, an imprint of The Haworth Press, Inc.) Vol. 25, No. 3/4, 2006, pp. 197-221; and: *Faith-Based Social Services: Measures, Assessments, and Effectiveness* (ed: Stephanie C. Boddie, and Ram A. Cnaan) The Haworth Pastoral Press, an imprint of The Haworth Press, Inc., 2006, pp. 197-221.

and Family. The challenges to data collection are presented and suggestions for doing participatory research in similar settings are discussed. doi:10.1300/J377v25n03_12

KEYWORDS. Faith-based programs, social welfare, participatory research designs, at-risk youth, charitable choice, and US Department of Health and Human Services, Administration for Children

The present Presidential Administration continues to strengthen the capacity of community and faith-based organizations to provide services among certain populations in the United States. Indeed, in the era of devolution to smaller providers, more faith-based providers have joined the competition for public funds. As such, there is an on-going need to evaluate the outcomes of the faith-based initiative and specific community based programs which utilize Compassion Capital grants.

This research was focused on a faith-based program during a time when the research community, funders and policy makers, were interested in rigorous evaluations of faith-based programs. These stakeholders and others, including the public at large, seek to separate conjecture and reality in understanding whether faith-based services offer unique benefits or risks to participants. These developments have given voice to concerns about faith based providers' professionalism and capacity. On one hand, the lure of community and faith-based provision of services is their access to marginalized populations (Verba, Scholzman, & Brady, 1995; Wuthnow, Hackett, & Hsu, 2004); unique resources, and potential cost-effectiveness (Campbell et al., 2003; Cnaan & Boddie, 2001; Kennedy & Bielefeld, 2003). On the other hand, though the research has not necessarily borne out all the following, a number of concerns have been raised about smaller faith-based providers': capacity issues, including needs for structured record keeping systems, complying with government standards, or additional funding (Kramer, Finegold, De Vita, & Wherry, 2005); respect for the religious freedom of participants, fiscal accountability, sustainability, or level of professionalism (Jeavons, 2003; Lewis, 2003), fewer technical and financial resources (Jeavons, 2003; Lewis, 2003, Rock, 2002).

Studies of faith-based social services have confirmed that the need for technical support, additional funding, and record keeping capabilities. Participatory research approaches can help build capacity. Thus, participatory methods are an appropriate choice to evaluate community-based programs, such as many smaller faith-based programs. Participatory research designs are distinguished by their intentional collaboration with "clients" as research participants in evaluating the project or initiative. Participatory research has been traditionally used within historically disenfranchised populations since it allows participants to have more control, gain access to resources, and develop skills in critical evaluation, problem-solving and decision-making (Zimmerman, Israel, Schulz, & Checkoway, 1992). The evaluation is viewed as a vehicle to empower the community, program, or program participants to facilitate, assess, and contribute to the change they wish to enact. While participatory approaches have been more commonly used outside of the U.S., this approach has gained momentum in the U.S. since the late 1980s. The Government Performance and Results Act of 1993 stipulated that grantees be involved as key participants in implementation (Atkinson, Wilson, & Avula, (2005). Such changes call for sophistication of participatory evaluation methods (Mott, 2003, Weiss, 2003).

A second reason for using participatory models when studying faith-based providers is a value shared by social work and religion in general–that of social transformation. Healy (2001) points to Lewen's work on theory of action, as well as the work of Paulo Freire, Gramsci, Marx, and Engels, as setting precedent for participatory action research's (PAR) role in social transformation. Likewise, the most popular religions of the world share a commitment to the betterment of the individual, serving others who are in need, and promoting peace within societies. It must be noted that within every religious tradition, small subsets of zealous members may interpret their religion in such a way to promote violence, but this is often not the majority view within that religion.

Healy (2001) has critiqued much of what has come to be labeled PAR in the U.S.–suggesting that often, PAR designs within social work research do not rigorously maintain their reformative tenets. This highlights the divergent goals of advocacy and research. Having noted Healy's critique, suffice it to say that given the constraints of time, money, and personnel, this case study did not attempt to carry out "rigorous" PAR. However, the study utilized participatory methods and this decision influenced the data collection.

The case study was participatory in that the evaluation was initiated not by an external researcher, but by the program's oversight committee. Program staff and youth participants were involved in planning, data collection, analysis, and dissemination of results. In addition, one of the major goals of the research-practice partnership was to gain first-hand insight to the experiences of urban minority youth, youth at risk, and practitioners, and to add their voices to the public discourse about youth and community development and publicly-funded faith-based endeavors. The decision to have staff carry out some research activities was agreed to by the lead pastor and key administrative personnel, but this did not prevent "glitches" in the data collection. In other words, while there was no outward reluctance from staff to be involved in data collection and analysis, but programmatic demands on staff time, lack of computers and office space, changes in personnel, and the evolving environment of the program contributed to delays in data collection and loss of data.

All of these issues come into play when deciding the best design to evaluate community-based and faith-based programs. While research on faith-based programs has increased since the passage of the Charitable Choice legislation, demands for "faith factor" research which is more rigorous and empirical may clarify the content, processes, and diversity within faith-based service implementation and outcomes, and thus inform research. For example, despite the growing acceptance of religiosity as a multidimensional factor, it is more common for studies to use less complex measures such as religious affiliation or attendance at religious activities to assess individual religiosity. However, measuring individual religiosity in a more sensitive manner is a challenge: appropriate methods and instruments for evaluating the range of impact or interactions that may be connected to religion and which take into account the multidimensional nature of private and organized religion, are needed (Sinha, Cnaan, Jones, & Dichter, 2003; Smith, 2003). In order to assess youths' religiosity, this case study used the 32-item Multidimensional Measure of Religiousness/Spirituality which included questions about how often the youths' family prays over a meal, youths' sense of closeness to God, and frequency of attendance at worship and other religious activities (Fetzer Institute, 1999). In addition, youth were asked background questions about their families' attendance at a congregation, and during interviews and focus groups, about their personal beliefs and attitude toward religion.

A second methodological concern is how to measure such factors as the content, integration, and application of religious components in a faith-based program. In other words, how can the presence and the extent to which strictly religious elements are implicitly or overtly expressed during service provision, be assessed (Fisher, 2003; Kramer,

Finegold, De Vita, & Wherry, 2005; Sider & Unruh, 2004; Smith & Sosin, 2001)? This is important given the wide range of programs which fall under the title "faith-based," and the various ways that the programs implement their services. For example, some programs may have been started by a congregation or religious group but have become religious "in name only" over time: virtually no part of their service provision may contain a religious element. In an overview of welfare to work programs in four cities, Monsma and Mounts (2002) found that less than two-fifths reported explicit religious elements in their services. Other programs incorporate elements into their service provision which could be considered religious. In order to triangulate data regarding the presence, frequency, and content of religious interactions within the program, this case study employed all of the following: participant observation, individual interviews with youth and staff in the program which asked them about religious elements, and a short questionnaire which asked participants to recall whether in the past 7 days, three types of potentially religious interactions had occurred.

Third, prior research largely confirms positive relationships between youth development and involvement in religious congregations (Blank & Davie, 2004; Donhue & Benson, 1995; Donelson, 1999; Sinha, Cnaan, & Gelles, 2005; Smith, 2005). It is logical to presume that faith-based programs can be an effective context in which to facilitate healthy development and socialization. However, research is needed to delineate whether faith-based *programs*, in addition to, or independently of religious involvement (such as being a part of a congregation), may impact participants. Only recently have researchers begun evaluating the role and impact of faith-based programs, as opposed to involvement in a religious congregation, in youth interventions (White & de Marcellus, 1998). This case study design offered an opportunity to address the question of whether participation in a faith-based program, *as opposed to religious congregations*, was related to positive impacts for youth. Through surveys and interviews, youths' involvement in religious activities and congregations was assessed. Then, youth who were regularly engaged in religious congregations and those who were not could be compared on a number of responses. In addition to involvement in a religious congregation, this study assessed other background variables to strengthen the study's internal validity (Yegidis & Weinbach, 2002).

In response to these concerns, the mixed-method case study design offered methodological innovation: a naturalistic setting was observed through combined qualitative and quantitative methods to allow triangulation of multidimensional data from various sources. This article offers lessons learned from a participatory research approach for a federally-funded, 10-month mixed-methods case study of a faith- and community-based alternative education program for youth. I present here a few key findings from the study and then briefly describe the program. Next, I reflect on the challenges encountered during data collection and offer suggestions for addressing them in future research.

DESCRIPTION OF THE PROGRAM

The program studied was an alternative education program for truant, at risk, and other youth aged 14-21. The youth in the program could be characterized as being among the highest risk in the region. Youth were either referred from city's Department of Human Services (DHS) Truancy Prevention department, or voluntarily attended the program rather than attend a public school or other disciplinary educational institution. The case study assessed change in youths' behaviors and attitudes as well as youth's perceptions of the program, whether religious elements were implemented in the program, and program impact using a combination of surveys, interviews, and participant observation. To give the reader a sense of the program, I will briefly describe its origin and what the program was like during the data collection period.

The alternative education program originated within one congregation when their welfare to work program, which served primarily women, began attracting younger clients seeking education and job training in the late 1990s. Supported by a grant from a local city agency, this congregation began educating, mentoring, and counseling high-risk teens who had dropped out of other traditional educational programs. The 35 teens who entered the program were characterized by: being truant; one third has offended, one-fourth had used or sold drugs, had reading skills ranging from the 2nd to the 4th grade, one third were parents or had been pregnant; a third had mental health issues; four had received public assistance and nine had been homeless.

In 2002, the lead congregation began expanding the education program in collaboration with seven other congregations. The congregations had a shared heritage: they were of the same denomination, race, and were located in a close proximity in the city. As a group, the congregations applied for and received funding through the youth services and truancy prevention department of the city's Department of Human Services (DHS). In 2005, the program continues to serve more than 60 youth. In addition to providing alternative education, six of the eight congregations opened teen lounges for community youth where teens could relax, do homework, play games such as pool, video games, basketball, or work on a computer during varying afternoon, evening, or weekend hours. Older youth and adults from the congregation monitored the lounge use. In addition to community youth, youth in the education program were invited to use the teen lounges.

The alternative education component consisted of a Monday through Friday, 9am to 3pm, program that took place in three churches located within 2 miles of each other. Classroom instruction in core subjects–math, science, English, and social studies was supplemented with instruction in other subjects including computer and software skills, music, art, drama, entrepreneurship, and life skills. The program was organized into six-week sessions separated by a no-class week during which staff re-organized and planned the next six-week session. Youth in the program received formal and informal counseling from staff, teachers, pastors, a licensed therapist, and case management from Master's level social workers. Credits earned in the alternative program counted toward a high school diploma from a neighborhood high school. The program encompassed students with varied learning support needs, and was flexible enough to make its day to day schedule conducive to students' situations: some students had work or family responsibilities that restricted their available hours during the day. These students could work on units at home (such as a math chapter or book report) and come in weekly to meet with an instructor.

Combined, the Teen Lounge and education components were carried out by more than two dozen individuals. Paid staff included: an executive director, a program administrator, three site coordinators, one education coordinator, two full-time and several part-time teachers, two masters level social workers, an outreach and recruitment person, a curriculum development consultant, and a part-time licensed therapist. Other staff and volunteers included three building maintenance or janitorial staff, two secretaries, a pastor who thrice-daily chauffeured students from site to site, and a handful of congregation members who prepared lunches for students. Not all staff were full-time and not all were compensated from the DHS grant: some volunteered and some were paid from congregation budgets.

There were no formal religious components to the program. Youth were not asked to participate in prayer, or any religious teaching such as a devotional or scripture study as part of the regular 9am to 3pm program. The program name was not religious in nature. Youth were told that the program was faith-based, but during the orientation, youth were informed of that all faiths were respected at the program and that there were no mandatory religious elements during the program. Students signed a waiver indicating that they understood this. On the other hand, the program was held in three church buildings, youth were transported in a church van which was driven by a pastor, and all the staff members were active members in their congregations. The executive director was also pastor of the lead church and staff and students alike called her "Pastor."

Other religious influences in the program were by invitation only. For example, youth who used the education program or the teen lounges might be invited to activities that the churches held, such as Bible Studies, retreats, movie nights, basketball tournaments, dances, and other special events. The staff were instructed to be respectful of all faith traditions and students' "faith" in general. The exutive director told me, "we respect faith. We are faith-sensitive." Earlier, the lead church's welfare to work program complied with one Muslim woman's desire to pray by giving her adequate space, privacy, and time to pray during the day.

Given the impromptu social events planned by congregations, the six-week rotating subject schedule, and the flexibility of the program model to respond to varying interests and resources among the youth, staff, volunteers, and budget, the program was a constantly evolving entity. (Now in its third year, many of these fluctuations have evened out.) During the ten months of data collection, the program expanded from one primary site with 35 students housed in one congregation to three sites with over 60 students which were supervised by the collaborative of congregations, oversight for the program gradually shifted from the primary lead congregation to the leadership committee of the cluster of congregations. The transition involved hiring new staff and redefining existing job positions and responsibilities.

The staff continued to refine organizational processes to facilitate communication and consistency within and across sites. Mid way through the first year of expanded operation, for example, staff spent many hours during the no-class week reforming processes to monitor student attendance, academic progress, the curriculum, transportation needs, the program schedule, and solidifying such procedures as: how to cancel a class, how to prevent and respond to unusual occurrences such as a fight between students, and reviewing the employee manual (personal communication, January 14, 2004). The evolution included student turnover as well: initially, students entered and then left the education component due to various reasons such as a change in residence, "dropping out," entering other programs such as Job Corp, or being incarcerated. This created a sense of flux in the program population. Over time, other staff and students formed a stable core.

Other issues were related to the "expansion" stage of the program's development. Student transportation, providing student lunches, heating old buildings with old boilers in a very cold winter, DHS payment delays, and occasional delays of payroll occurred. In addition, at times, lack of additional computers, reliable copiers and printers, and office supplies such as paper, pens, folders, and filing cabinets affected daily operations. Staff and congregations volunteered their own supplies, vehicles, paint, money, volunteers, and building maintenance to keep the program operating smoothly. Thus, while the program was not entirely new during the data collection, many aspects of the program were modified. The impact of the "start-up/expansion" nature of the expanding program on this case study cannot be overstated.

These examples serve to introduce the factors which affected the data collection process. On the positive side, the warmth of program staff and students and their willingness to participate in the research offered tremendous benefits in terms of accessibility to students, staff, and data. This willingness to engage in evaluation has been noted as a characteristic of faith-based organizations (Trulear, 2000). In addition, amicable relationships and pleasurable site visits made the work delightful even when collecting data was tedious. The following section discusses in detail the challenges which were encountered during the ten-month data collection period and how they were addressed.

KEY FINDINGS

A few of the key findings of the study are as follows. The study assessed youth's self-reported change in four areas: peer and key relationships, use of free time, educational goals, and religiosity. In addition, the study assessed whether youths with more and less prior religious involvement (such as attending a congregation frequently) responded differently to the survey after spending time in the program.

One of the most important findings of this study was that youth who attend faith-based programs which provide a "secular" service, such as education did not find the program "religious." In particular, while youth described the staff as "religious," they did not perceive the program as religious and were not uncomfortable attending the program in a church building.

One of the most helpful findings of the study was that the program succeeded in creating an atmosphere that was safe for students. It is quite likely that a combination of things fostered this positive environment. There were a smaller number of students, with a maximum of about 65 students at a given time. Positive peer dynamics were expected and modeled by the staff and by younger "peer" counselors who volunteered with the program. The program staff were dedicated to treating each student as a responsible adult who had to choose whether they would take advantage of the learning opportunities the program. In other words, the program did not have a "punitive" disciplinary framework. If a student chose to goof around or talk during classtime rather than utilize this time to study or work, they could. One result was that some students didn't work on their independent curriculum as quickly as they could. This was sometimes a distraction for other students, but it also gave the program a "fun" atmosphere that was attractive to many students who had failed to progress at traditional institutions. Students were allowed to progress at their own pace–however slow or fast this was. Despite a sometimes chaotic atmosphere, one of the most frequent observations of students was that they liked being able to work at their own pace and they liked being able to get individualized attention when they needed it from instructors.

Youth repeatedly mentioned their appreciation of this individualized attention–for both academic and personal issues. Youth trusted the staff and felt staff cared for them. Unlike other education environments, youth felt safe at the program and were better able to form friendships with other youth. The lack of fights which occurred in the program context was a striking contrast to youths' descriptions of their prior experiences in public school or disciplinary schools.

The high rate of youths' attendance in the program was a marked change given that many had been truant or skipped school often prior to joining the program. Interviewed youth reported less time spent "hanging out," "running the streets," or "skipping class" than before entering the program, and some youth participated in other activities offered in connection with a congregation.

In terms of religiosity, the study showed mixed results. First, despite the fact that youth did not view the education program as "religious," survey results indicated that about half of the time, surveyed staff and youth remembered praying, talking about something religious, or being invited to a religious activity in the previous seven days. However, most youth reported no impact of the program on their personal religious beliefs and behaviors. Second, the survey data confirmed that youth who were more frequently involved with a religious congregation also had families who were more involved; spent more time in religious activities; felt they "worked with God as a partner" more often; and read scripture more frequently than youth who were least involved in a religious congregation. Finally, *only* youth who attended a congregation least (less than twice a month) showed an increase in how often they "worked with God as a partner" and in how often they reported attending any religious activity.

Challenges Encountered During Data Collection

Given that the program spanned three sites, was in an expansion stage, engaged more than two dozen staff and volunteers, and involved youth who had failed at other educational institutions, implementing data collection procedures was not readily or quickly achieved. The case study design included all youth who used the teen lounges or education component of the program during the 10-month data collection period. Study participants were recruited on a rolling basis by program staff during their orientation to the program and by youth counselors when they voluntarily came to the Teen Lounges.

Data was gathered through interviews and focus groups, surveys, and participant observation to assess change in: youths' use of free time; educational and vocational aspirations; identity and well-being; and religiosity. Issues which impeded or prevented data collection are discussed here according to the data source.

Interviews and Focus Groups

A sub sample of 20 youth was interviewed for about an hour. The semi-structured, open-ended interview covered the topics of: youths' background, experience of the program, religious environment of the program, family religious background, and influences on youth by their friends, adults and others in their lives. In particular, students' were asked about their prior education experience, if they had been truant, how they used their time if they had been truant, personal goals and aspirations, and whether they felt that being in the program had made a difference in their aspirations and self valuation. I began to follow up with students' answers about their previous educational experiences–which, without exception included involvement in fights with other students or with teachers. As will be discussed later, when another data source was unavailable, this additional information from the one-on-one interviews became important to assess youths' success and behavior changes related to peer and key relationships.

The original design was to select students randomly from the total list of enrolled students. Several practical issues necessitated using convenience sampling for the interview sub sample instead of random sampling. First, enrollment in the program was on-going, which negated getting a full list of students. Second, youth could only be contacted through the program–that is, the researcher did not have access to contact information for youth. However, even for program staff, contacting students at home was a tedious process given that some students did not have answering machines, messages might not be passed along, and some students stayed at more than one address. Thus, youth were contacted during weekly site visits and interviews were scheduled for the following weeks. I met with students over the lunch hour and provided lunch. Students were compensated for their time in the interview. Once set up, this scheduling process worked well and rarely did students not show up for the interview.

Focus groups were conducted at three sites. The focus groups were scheduled with youth from the congregation who monitored the teen lounges. Participants were asked about their use of the Teen Lounge, their relationship to the congregation, and questions from the individual interview questionnaire, including the youth's view of religion, their family's religious background, and about whether and how youth integrate religious components into their lives. Youth were compensated for their time. The original design was to conduct 2 focus groups at each site and up to 8 sites were expected to be open by the end of the data collection.

A number of issues impacted the number of focus groups that were conducted. First was the rate at which the teen lounges opened. At the outset of the data collection period, two Teen Lounges were open, and four additional lounges opened over the 10-month data collection period. Though six lounges were officially open at some point during the data collection period, only half of the lounges were used regularly by community youth. At two lounges, problems with the heating systems meant lounges were unheated and unused for several months. At another congregation, the lounge opened several months into the data collection period and the lounge was not used by community youth as planned. Twice, a focus group at this site was scheduled and cancelled due to conflict with other building uses and lack of youth. At a fourth congregation, the lounge was not being used by community youth, but served as a gathering place for church youth group meetings.

These practical developments–from cold weather to lounges not being used as expected, affected the number of focus groups that could be conducted. In order to gain sufficient information about how the lounges were being used, informal follow-up observations at five of the open lounges were conducted.

Religiosity Survey

A multidimensional survey of religiousness/spirituality was used to assess background factors for youth religiosity and youth's self-reported religious behavior and attitudes. The religiosity survey covered a range of topics such as attendance at religious services, finding strength in religion, perception of congregation's support, and a brief spiritual history. The survey was piloted and slight modifications were made from the original survey produced by the NIA/Fetzer Institute (Fetzer Institute, 1999). The religiosity survey was administered by a classroom instructor to youth during class time after they entered the education component. Youth who did not participate in the education component of the program were given the survey during youth meetings and focus groups. As many as possible youth who remained active in the program at least four weeks after they entered it were given the survey a second time. Of the 73 youth who filled out the religiosity survey initially, 36 youth filled out the survey a second time.

It was difficult to implement a consistent routine which ensured that youth took the survey early on in the program. In other words, due to the flexible and staggered nature of the program's initial assessment period, some students were not given the survey (by their class instructor) immediately upon enrollment. The average time that youth spent in the program before taking the survey the first time was 12 weeks. Student attendance habits added to the teacher's difficulty in administering the survey: though student attendance was quite consistent, (averaging more than three days a week), fewer students came to class in a timely, "full-day" fashion, which meant teachers had to remember from day to day who had taken the survey. In addition, teachers could have new students almost weekly. These factors affected teachers' ability to track who had taken the survey. Teachers were willing but obtaining the surveys required frequent follow-up. In the end, despite the plan for students to take the religiosity survey the week they entered the program, this often did not occur.

This was true for collecting the survey from youth who used teen lounges as well. Most teen lounge youth were given the religiosity survey when they participated in a focus group, and this did not necessarily correspond to when they started using the lounge. This was due in part to the inconsistent use of the lounges over the winter months. Many youth could not be contacted (through the lounges) to do a follow-up religiosity survey. All of these factors diminished the ability of the survey to capture potential change in youths' responses. That is, since it was not administered to students as soon as they entered the program, the survey results were less likely to capture the full range of change.

Observation Checklist

In addition to the religiosity survey, a short 4-question survey called the Observation Checklist was developed to gather information on the content and frequency of religious elements that voluntarily occurred during the program. Based on the typology of implicit and explicit religious components at faith-based programs from the work of Sider and Unruh (2002), the Checklist assessed whether, in the past 7 days, a respondent initiated or observed prayer, discussed spiritual or religious matters, or voluntarily attended a religious event connected with a congregation. Respondents were anonymous but were asked to identify their position in the program such as "student," "staff," "teacher," "social worker," or "pastor."

The Observation Checklist was to be collected non-systematically, but frequently, to ensure a good representation. The original data collection plan was to have a staff person and teachers hand out and collect these short surveys during meetings and during class. This plan did not work. Getting surveys to and from the staff and teachers, and getting them filled out on a weekly basis never occurred for a number of reasons: there wasn't a central place to leave the blank survey forms, surveys that were left in a mailbox would not get retrieved; or staff and teachers would forget to hand out and collect the surveys during meetings and class. The only effective method was that I carried survey forms with me and every time I visited a site, I would hand out the forms to any staff and youth who could fill them out immediately and hand them back to me. The forms took only about one minute to fill out.

In the end analysis, fewer observation checklists were collected than planned. Rather than using the observation checklist to capture fluctuation in voluntary religious interactions over time, the checklists could only confirm that on average, about 50 percent of the surveys reported some type of religious interaction in the previous seven days.

"CASI" Interview

Another source of data was a diagnostic assessment interview called the Comprehensive Adolescent Severity Index (CASI) which was administered by program social workers. The decision to have social workers administer the CASI was a direct result of the commitment to a participatory design. The research funds covered the cost of the CASI software and training so that the staff would gain the skills and capacity to have a long-term, "built-in" assessment tool for the program. The CASI is a 45-90 minute, semi-structured, clinical assessment and outcomes interview designed for repeat administration. The CASI assesses 10 life areas for youth, including education level and history; use of free time; peer and family relationships; social support; and mental health history. The CASI's automated data collection system (C-CASI) enabled direct entry of data during the semi-structured interview and included immediate validation and consistency checks (Meyers et al., 1998). The CASI was the primary instrument to assess youths' change over time in the four key areas of the study: peer and key relationships; use of free time; educational/vocational goals, and mental health. However, the social workers were only able to complete 30 initial CASIs and no follow up CASIs were conducted with youth after they had been in the program for at least three months. Several combined and uncontrollable events contributed to the poor collection of the CASI survey and the resulting lack of CASI data, including not enough trained staff to conduct the survey, faulty equipment, and not having a secure location for the computer which housed the CASI software.

First, though the program employed MSW-level social workers who received training to conduct the CASI, staffing changes and adjusting to the program's rapid expansion left the social workers with many responsibilities. The program employed one to two social workers at a time. The early months of data collection coincided with the program receiving newly enrolled youth. At that time, only one CASI-trained social worker was employed full time and conducted the CASI with five youth. In a few months time, a second social worker was employed part time and conducted two CASI interviews. Shortly thereafter, this social worker was diagnosed with an advanced illness and was not able to continue her employment. Approximately two months passed before she was replaced and a new social worker was trained to conduct the CASI. This third social worker was employed part time and conducted eight CASI surveys in a two-month period.

In addition to the limits of the social worker's availability, another mishap occurred. The computer where the CASI was installed at the primary site was not in a secure location, but "floated" on a moveable stand and was used by several staff members. Several months into the data collection period, this computer crashed and information stored on the hard drive was irrecoverable. The CASI software was installed on a computer at the second site and the social worker transported youth from one site to the second site to conduct the CASI.

During the cold winter months, the office with the second CASI-installed computer could not be heated. The computer had to be shifted to a warmer part of the building. The computer was moved from its secure location in a locked office, to a classroom. The classroom was used for multiple purposes, including an afterschool program, Sunday School, and church meetings. This meant that many people had access to the computer. At some point, the CASI software on this computer was tampered with and the data stored became irretrievable. Although we consulted with CASI developer and attempted several ways of copying and transferring the CASI data from this hard drive, the software had been changed and we were not able to access it. At the end of the data collection period, only 8 CASI interviews were available of the 30 which had been conducted.

Though the CASI data had been planned as the primary data source on changes in youths' relationships, educational aspiration, and certain mental health items, there were too few CASI interviews available to make the information useful. As previously noted, loss of the CASI data necessitated using a number of items from the religiosity survey as well as information from the interviews and focus groups to confirm findings about youths' peer and key relationships; use of free time; educational/vocational goals, and mental health.

Of all the tactical issues brought forth in the case study, the failure to collect and store the CASI data speaks most to the type of capacity issues that have been raised as concerns when studying informal programs such as some faith-based ones. First, this program had computers, but the computers were quite old and less reliable. The congregations did not have cash on hand to purchase new equipment, nor did they have enough computers to designate some for program use. Instead, not only computers, but office and classroom space were used for church purposes as well. This meant that the data's security was compromised.

A second capacity issue was around staffs' responsibilities. Staff clearly had the necessary professional qualifications. However, since a number of staff were part time, they could not easily fulfill their social work duties and implement the diagnostic CASI interview. This became particularly noticeable because of the participatory nature of the design in which program equipment and space were used to carry out research activities.

It is likely that staffing responsibilities would have "ironed themselves out" over time as the social workers' workload and office space became more consistent and the student enrollment evened out. On the other hand, the technical glitches which prevented the security of the collected CASI interviews are more likely to represent continued challenges to data collection and participatory research. This raises an important consideration for the evaluation of smaller programs in general. Without additional funding, programs will not have the technological capacity to easily collect, store, analyze, and present data. In this case study, the lack of funding for computers and other helpful technological advances such as Web-based data collection, resulted in irretrievable data losses. If stakeholders, such as the faith-based initiative and researchers, are sincere in wanting to accurately evaluate and increase the capacity of such programs, then funding for technological advances and up-to-date equipment is paramount.

Participant Observation

Participant observation occurred at the following types of events during the data collection period: program staff meetings and administrative meetings; "class" time and informal observations at the three education sites during program hours; teen lounges; youth meetings; conversations with various program personnel, volunteers, and representatives from the funding agency; phone conversations with various staff; cluster meetings; cluster-wide planning events; community lectures at congregation sites; religious services; social events organized for youth by the program or by a congregation. Handwritten or typed notes were taken during or shortly after these events and conversations and were coded for analysis. Documents collected for analysis included meeting minutes, e-mail and written communications, the original program manual, newsletters, and program brochures.

The informal and face-to-face communication culture of the program was both a bane and an advantage for carrying out participant observation. On one hand, as a researcher who was not on site daily, I had difficulty at times finding out when meetings were being held or when schedules had changed. While the staff who were at the program daily relied on word of mouth communication, the researcher is often, and in this case, unintentionally, left out of the loop. Getting certain documents, such as meeting minutes or program records, also took time. While the administrators of the program was always willing to work with me, it usually took several reminders, several months, and a few face-to-face meetings before I could obtain copies. I respect the demands on staff time, and the low priority of passing along certain documents given other far more pressing and important tasks. However, at times the patience and persistence needed to get certain kinds of information frustrated the efficiency of data collection.

On the other hand, staff and youth always welcomed my presence and spoke with me informally whenever I was on site. I occasionally "walked into" a meeting or class unannounced and was always welcomed. Thus, my access to every day occurrences and informal face to face interactions was almost limitless. This leads me to believe that I was privy to a very candid observation of the program and its daily reality.

LESSONS LEARNED

In numerous public forums and in published materials, the role of faith-based organizations in providing publicly funded services has been debated. Debate topics spurred by increased public funding for faith-based and religious social service providers include their capacity, their effectiveness, and whether they make unique contributions to the welfare mix. How to appropriately evaluate faith-based services and whether to use strictly outcome-based measures have been raised. This article examined the data collection process during a federally-funded intensive case study at one collaborative faith-based program using participatory methods. This section presents some practical lessons for studying small community-based and faith-based programs when a participatory approach is desirable.

Interviews

During interviews, the use of follow-up questions and extra question was used to explore other topics. Though it took more time and resulted in longer interviews, the data provided valuable insights to students' lives and was helpful when the CASI data source was not available. In addition, scheduling interviews on-site with youth worked far better than going through a receptionist or staff. It is possible that the added incentive of a lunch and compensation, youth were highly motivated to come for their interview. By far, one of the most enjoyable aspects of the research were these one-on-one interviews with youth: youth were candid, didn't mind being tape recorded and were respectful, intelligent, and insightful.

Focus Groups

The planned number of focus groups could not be implemented due to inconsistent start up rates and inconsistent use of the teen lounges. Alternatively, data collection switched to less formal observation as opposed to scheduled focus group discussions. The inconsistent use of the teen lounges at two of the sites was related to the cost of fixing broken boilers. One of the concerns that has been raised in broader discussion is about the "technical capacity" of smaller or less formal providers. Though the congregations generously brought all their resources to the table, including their physical space, the congregation buildings were older and some needed updates to electrical wiring, infrastructure, window replacement, heating system, and phone/cable lines to facilitate more phone lines and faster Internet access. When the heating systems failed in the two main sites, it affected the program atmosphere substantially. While the program itself was not interrupted, adjustments such as shifting the location of classes, postponing teen lounge activities, and relying on alternate sources of heat were required.

A notable aspect of this discussion about physical capacity is that despite the cold temperatures and loudness of the work space, students continued to come regularly. As one staff member put it, . . . "why are [the youth] here?" He said, "It's loud, it's cold [inside!], there's no food"– they have to bring their own or go buy lunch. His answer? "Relationships." Relationships are the only thing he can think of that keeps them coming here–here they get a friendly hello, they interact with friends, and staff and teacher. The warmth is not temporal but emotional (NPC-CUNorman-chat22Jan04, Paragraph 19).

While the "warmth" of relationships does not occur exclusively in faith-based or small programs, the importance of this quality, and its effect in contrast to physical capacities, should not be overlooked.

Religiosity Survey

One major data collection challenge was getting the survey collected as soon as possible after students enrolled in the program. While the expectations of staff and the motive of following a participatory action research model meant involving the teachers as the primary collection agent for the survey, given the demands on the teachers' time, the evolving nature of the student body, and changes in the program during its first year of expansion, the survey was not administered in as timely a fashion as desired. Hindsight suggests that there was no other staff person who could have regularly administered the surveys, so that resorting to a (non-program) researcher would have been necessary to ensure that surveys were handed out and collected in a timely fashion. This would have lessened the participatory role of the teachers in the research but would have resulted in getting the religiosity survey collected closer to students' entrance into the program and might have been reflected in more significant changes in the survey responses over time.

Observation Checklist

Similar to the religiosity survey, the challenge with collecting the Observation Checklist was getting surveys handed out and collected in a timely fashion. The original plan had been to collect Checklists non-systematically, but weekly, by staff and teachers. However, there was not enough routine established at the program during this year of expansion for staff and teachers to easily implement this survey on a weekly basis. Instead, the Checklist was handed out and immediately collected by the researcher during site visits. However practical this method, there were limits: the primary site was visited most frequently (about weekly) but the other sites were visited less frequently. While the Checklist was a very useful tool in terms of recording the occurrence of and type of religious activities that took place during the program, it would work best in settings whose daily activities occurred more routinely than this particular program. *Participant Observation*–On a few occasions, information about when and where meetings were going to be held was not passed along in a timely fashion. This did not appear to be any intentional exclusion, but rather that most of the program staff were present enough for word-of-mouth communication to be effective. Conversely, the informality of the program setting, and the staff's willingness to participate fully in the case study, provided the researcher with easy and usually immediate access to meetings, classroom settings, informal conversations and phone calls. The staff and students were extremely pleasant and willing to work with any request presented.

HINDSIGHT AND FORESIGHT: CONCLUDING THOUGHTS

This case study presents a number of practical applications for researchers who are evaluating smaller or less formal programs, including those which are faith- and community-based. First, the use of mixed methods and triangulating data sources was helpful for assessing the impact of the program. When the CASI data was not available for analysis, the religiosity survey and interview transcripts provided much of the information needed to assess the research questions. Second, researchers who maintain a flexible and creative approach to data collection may be better able to adjust and take advantage of available sources of data that were not originally planned. For example, taking the time to ask extra and follow-up questions during individual interviews provided insight to students' prior education backgrounds and their perceptions of the program, particularly the religious aspects. Third, researchers who do case studies in naturalistic settings and who choose to involve participants in the research must have patience and endurance for the inevitable glitches which will occur. In this case, acknowledging the stresses incurred by program staff and which affected the data collection, also led me to admire and respect how the staff showed up cheerfully each day despite: occasionally delayed paychecks; a less-than-market pay rate; students' personal situations and interactions which were sometimes tragic and often frustrating; lack of employee benefits through the program; lack of amenities such as a warm office, coffee, or ample paper and copier supplies. Acknowledging the realities of the expanding program and of staff's other responsibilities made not getting a survey in on time easy to understand.

Mott (2003) suggested that participatory evaluations sidestep the lack of trust and perceived lack of relevance or value that sometimes occur in external evaluations. Staff who understand and participate in evaluative activities gain a sense of ownership of the data and the ability to assess themselves. Having a good relationship with the leaders and staff of the program helped immensely. I had almost unrestricted access to classrooms, meetings, and staff opinions. The willingness of staff to participate in the research may have also made it easier for the youth to trust me and to be willing to take the surveys and be candid during interviews. Without the support of the staff, it may have been more difficult to get the youth's participation and to collect as many surveys and interviews. The participation was meaningful rather than the often token participation/partnership with faith-based groups.)

Participatory action research is an important niche in the realm of social services evaluation. In general, social service evaluation has been seen as the cutting edge of social science research both in the U.S. and in international settings (Boruch, 1994; Mott, 2003). Not only can participatory approaches to evaluation build the capacity of the organization being studied, but also afford the organization more ownership of the process, visibility in the local setting and with funders, and legitimizes its program results. In this case, the research funding enabled a number of staff to go through the training for the CASI interview, which heightened their awareness of the potential risks and difficulties youth in this population may be facing, and gave staff an opportunity to discuss how best to respond to these issues before they arose with any student. The CASI software was purchased and licensed through the research funding and the program continues to use this diagnostic tool as a way to assess youth and track their progress. The program director also decided to include a few questions about youths' faith in the CASI interview as a way to ascertain whether this was perceived as a strength for any youth, as well as to track change in youth's faith over time.

There are also many practical challenges to doing participatory action research within naturalistic settings, including: high turnover of staff or program beneficiaries (Fisher, 2003); designing methods which can be successfully implemented; and limited technical resources (Fisher, 2003; Johnson, Tompkins, & Webb, 2002). Researchers who want to undertake research with worthwhile results should consider how to include funding for up to date computers, new technology, office supplies, support for staff to complete the research tasks, and staff training. Making sure that staff understand the time and resource requirements of the research and are fully supportive is necessary.

The benefits of participatory research in a naturalistic setting are ethical and empowering: the voices of participants and practitioners are amplified as evaluators of their own program and interpreters of their own data (Fawcett et al., 1996; Myers, 2003; Sinha & Cnaan, 2004). One of the ways this occurred during this case study was through individual interviews with youth and reporting the youth's positive and negative perceptions back to staff. Staff also provided important interpretive feedback when youths' responses to a survey question changed in an unexpected direction. During participatory research, staff gain useful skills in self and program assessment (Mott, 2003), multiple levels of organizational data and analysis can be facilitated (Myers, 2003), and unexpected insights can occur. The challenge for researchers, as pointed out by Fisher (2003) is to balance the need for rigorous research design while engaging local participants fully and obtaining measures which are meaningful to various stakeholders.

REFERENCES

Atkinson, D. D., Wilson, M., & Avula, D. (2005). A participatory approach to building capacity of treatment programs to engage in evaluation. *Evaluation and Program Planning, 28*, 329-334.

Blank, S. & Davie, F. (2004, April) *Faith in their futures: The youth and congregations in partnership program of the Kings County (Brooklyn, NY)*. District Attorney's Office. Philadelphia, PA: Public Private Ventures.

Boruch, R. F. (1994). The future of controlled randomized experiments: A briefing. *Evaluation Practice, 15*(3), 265-274.

Campbell, D., Glunt, E., Bockman, S., Little, J., Nieman, M., & Sirotnik, B. W. (2003). Evaluating the California community and faith-based initiative. In The Independent Sector and The Roundtable on Religion and Social Welfare Policy, *The Role of Faith-Based Organizations in the Social Welfare System Working Papers* (pp. 181-194). Washington, DC: Independent Sector.

Cnaan, R. A., & Boddie, S. C. (2001). *Black church outreach: Comparing how Black and other congregations serve their needy neighbors*. Philadelphia, PA: University of Pennsylvania Center for Research on Religion and Urban Civil Society.

Fawcett, S., Paine-Andrews, A., Francisco, V. T., Schultz, J. A., Richter, K. P. Williams, E. L., Harris, K. J., Beri, C. M., & Fisher, J. L. (1996). Empowering community health initiatives through evaluation. In D. Fetterman & S. Kaftarian & Wandersman, A. (Eds.). *Empowerment Evaluation: Knowledge and tools for self-assessment and accountability* (pp. 161-187). Thousand Oaks, CA: Sage.

Fetzer Institute, (1999). *Multidimensional measurement of religiousness/spirituality for use in health research: A report of the Fetzer Institute on Aging Working Group*. Kalamazoo, MI: The Fetzer Institute.

Fischer, R. L. (2003). The devil is in the details: Implementing outcome measurement in faith-based organizations. Paper prepared for Independent Sector 2003 Spring Research Forum–The Role of Faith-Based Organizations in the Social Welfare System (January 2003). Bethesda, MD.

Healy, K. (2001). Participatory action research and social work: A critical appraisal. *International Social Work 44*(1), 93-105.

Hill, P. C., & Hood, R. W. (Eds.). (1999). *Measures of religiosity*. Birmingham, AL: Religious Education Press.

Jeavons, T. H. (2003). The Vitality and independence of religious organizations. *Society*, *40*(2), 27-36.

Johnson, B. R., Tompkins, R. B., & Webb, D. (2002). *Objective hope: Assessing the effectiveness of faith-based organizations: A review of the literature*. Center for Religion and Urban Civil Society. Philadelphia, PA: University of Pennsylvania.

Kennedy, S. S., & Bielefeld, W. (2003). *Charitable Choice: First results from three states*. Indianapolis, IN: Indiana University-Purdue University Indianapolis School for Public and Environmental Affairs, Center for Urban Policy and the Environment.

Kramer, F., Finegold, K., De Vita, C. J., & Wherry, L. (2005, July). *Federal policy on the ground: Faith-based organizations delivering local services*. Washington, DC: The Urban Institute.

Lewis, B. M. (2003). Issues and dilemmas in faith-based social service delivery: The case of the Salvation Army of Greater Philadelphia. *Administration in Social Work*, *27*, 87-106.

Meyers, K., Webb, A., Randall, M., McDermott, P., Mulvancy, F., Tucker, W., & McLellan, A.T. (1998) *Psychometric Properties of the Comprehensive Adolescent Severity Inventory (CASI)*. Paper presented at the 60th Annual Scientific Meeting of the College on Problems of Drug Dependence, Scottsdale, Arizona.

Monsma, S. V., & Mounts, C. M. (2002). *Working faith: How religious organizations provide welfare-to-work services*. Center for Religion and Urban Civil Society. Philadelphia, PA: University of Pennsylvania.

Mott, A. (2003). Hand in hand–Evaluation and organizational development. *The Evaluation Exchange*, *9*(3) [electronic version] Cambridge, MA: The Harvard Family Research Project. Retrieved January 14, 2005 from http://www.gse.harvard.edu/~hfrp/eval/issue23/index.html

Myers, V.L. (2003). Planning & Evaluating Faith-based Interventions: A Framework to Close the Theory Practice Divide. In *The Role of Faith-Based Organizations in the Social Welfare System: Working Papers*. Published by the Independent Sector & the Roundtable on Religion and Social Welfare Policy, Rockefeller Institute of Government: Albany New York.

Rock, J. (2002). *Stepping out on faith: New York City's Charitable Choice demonstration program*. Albany, NY: The Rockefeller Institute of Government, the Roundtable on Religion and Social Welfare Policy.

Sider, R., & Unruh, H. R. (2004). Commentary on typology of religious characteristics of social service and educational organizations and programs. *Nonprofit and Voluntary Sector Quarterly*, *33*, 135-139.

Sinha, J. W., & Cnaan, R. A. (2004). *Exploring the impact of a faith-based demonstration program for at-risk youth*. Washington, DC: Administration for Children and Families, Health and Human Services.

Sinha, J.W., Cnaan, R. A., & Gelles, R. (2005). *Is Religion Relevant for Teenagers? Impact of Religion on Risk Behavior*. Manuscript submitted for publication.

Sinha, J. W., Cnaan, R. A., Jones, D. L., & Dichter, S. (2003). Analysis of a collaborative faith-based demonstration project: The unique capacity of congregation- and community-based collaboration. In the Independent Sector *The Role of Faith-Based Organizations in the Social Welfare System Spring Research Forum: Working Papers* (pp. 159-168). Washington, DC: Independent Sector Roundtable on Religion and Social Welfare Policy.

Smith, C. (2005), *Soul Searching: The Religious and Spiritual Lives of American Teenagers.* New York: Oxford University Press

Smith, C. (2003). Theorizing religious effects among American adolescents. *Journal for the Scientific Study of Religion, 42*, 17-30.

Smith, S. R., & Sosin, M. R. (2001). *The varieties of faith-related agencies.* Public Administration Review, 61, 6, 651-670.

Verba, S., Schlozman, K. L., & Brady, H. E. (1995). *Voice and equality: Civic voluntarism in American politics.* Cambridge, MA: Harvard University.

Weiss, H. B. (2003). From the director's desk. *The Evaluation Exchange, 9*(3) [electronic version] Cambridge, MA: The Harvard Family Research Project. Retrieved January 14, 2005 from http://www.gse.harvard.edu/~hfrp/eval/issue23/index.html

White, J., & de Marcellus, M. (1998). *Faith-based outreach to at-risk youth in Washington, D.C.* Retrieved October 10, 2002 from Manhattan Institute: The Jeremiah Project Website http://www.manhattan-institute.org

Wuthnow, R., Hackett, C., & Hsu, B. Y. (2004). The effectiveness and trustworthiness of faith-based and other service organizations: A study of recipients' perceptions. *Journal for the Scientific Study of Religion, 43*, 1-18.

Yegidis, B., & Weinbach, R. (2002). *Research Methods for Social Workers.* Boston: Allyn and Bacon.

Zimmerman, M., Israel, B., Schulz, A., & Checkoway, B. (1992). Further explorations in empowerment theory: An empirical analysis of psychological empowerment. *American Journal of Community Psychology, 20*, 707-727.

Chapter 11

Evaluating the Effectiveness of Faith-Based Welfare Agencies: Methodological Challenges and Possibilities

Susan E. Grettenberger
John P. Bartkowski
Steven R. Smith

SUMMARY. This study examines the methodological challenges associated with conducting research on faith-based organizations. The arguments advanced are based on a group of comparative case studies conducted by the authors on secular and faith-based providers in three different social service domains: (1) transitional housing, (2) parent education, and (3) residential substance abuse treatment programs. All case studies utilized the same research protocol. The study identifies the lessons learned from comparative case study research on faith-based orga-

Susan E. Grettenberger, PhD, is Assistant Professor, Sociology, Anthropology, and Social Work (E-mail: grett1se@cmich.edu). John P. Bartkowski, PhD, is Professor of Sociology, Department of Sociology, Anthropology, & Social Work, PO Box C (USPS)/207 Bowen Hall (courier), Mississippi State University, Mississippi State, MS. Steven R. Smith, PhD, is Associate Dean and Director, Nancy Bell Evans Center on Nonprofits & Philanthropy, Daniel J. Evans School of Public Affairs, The University of Washington, Box 353055, Seattle, WA 98195.

[Haworth co-indexing entry note]: "Evaluating the Effectiveness of Faith-Based Welfare Agencies: Methodological Challenges and Possibilities." Grettenberger, Susan E., John P. Bartkowski, and Steven R. Smith. Co-published simultaneously in *Journal of Religion & Spirituality in Social Work* (The Haworth Pastoral Press, an imprint of The Haworth Press, Inc.) Vol. 25, No. 3/4, 2006, pp. 223-240; and: *Faith-Based Social Services: Measures, Assessments, and Effectiveness* (ed: Stephanie C. Boddie, and Ram A. Cnaan) The Haworth Pastoral Press, an imprint of The Haworth Press, Inc., 2006, pp. 223-240.

nizations when a similar protocol is implemented to examine a variety of social service domains and provider types. doi:10.1300/J377v25n03_13

KEYWORDS. Faith-based organizations, transitional housing, parent education, substance abuse programs, comparative case studies, charitable choice

Numerous assertions have been advanced concerning the benefits of services provided by faith-based organizations (FBOs), including claims about their superiority to secular nonprofits or government-run programs. These claims provided the basis for much of the initial support seen when the Bush administration first announced its plans to expand access to federal funding for faith-based organizations (Bush, 2001; Soskis, 2001). Many politicians, including President Bush, continue to advocate direct public funding of congregations and other faith-based organizations (FBOs) based on this presumption of superiority (Bush, 2005). Yet, insufficient research exists to support or dispute the claims being made about the effectiveness of FBO programs alone or in comparison to other programs (see Carlson-Theis, 2004; Chaves, 2004; DiIulio, 2004; Wuthnow, 2004).[1]

This study explores the methodological issues and challenges that emerge when research is conducted on faith-based organizations. The arguments offered here are based on a group of comparative case studies conducted by the authors. The authors contrasted secular and faith-based service agencies in three different social service domains, namely, transitional housing, parent education, and residential substance abuse treatment. In rendering a broad overview of these research projects, all of which utilized a similar protocol, this article identifies key methodological insights concerning research on FBOs and highlights a series of significant questions that require further investigation.

EVALUATING EFFECTIVENESS

There are two types of nonprofit program evaluation. The first type of nonprofit program evaluation is typically initiated by individual programs or agencies in response to what are now almost universal requirements by funders, accreditation bodies, and professional standards that document their program effectiveness (Morley, Vinson, & Hatry, 2001; Mulroy & Lauber, 2004; Herman & Renz, n.d.). Individual program evaluation also provides a feedback mechanism to the program planning process, feedback that allows improvement in a program's implementation and responsiveness to client need. The evaluation is a collaborative process, initiated and even implemented by the organization itself although it may work with a professional evaluator.

The second type of evaluation assesses social service programs and organizations more generally, answering broader questions about the effectiveness of a specific intervention or of programs within a service sector. Such evaluation has different purposes than does the program evaluation described above, purposes such as documenting best practices or informing policy decisions. Typically, the second type of research is conducted by an external, independent researcher. It is more formalized and rigorous research that seeks to assure a measure of control through its design, and allows for comparisons between different interventions or programs.

Single case studies using the latter approach are relatively common in a variety of program sectors (e.g., Mecca, Rivera, & Esposito, 2000; Somers & Piliawsky, 2004; Whipple & Nathans, 2005) and outcome studies of faith-based programs are just beginning to be completed (e.g., Rock, 2002). Comparative studies of different approaches to specific social problems are less common, while comparative studies of faith-based and nonreligious (that is, secular) services are still rare (e.g., Monsma & Mounts, 2002; Ragan, 2004). Yet, comparative studies that test claims about differences and the relative effectiveness of faith-based and secular programs are of great importance to the policy making process.

This paper seeks to encourage more comparative evaluations by discussing the challenges of evaluation research that compares FBOs and secular programs. This article is also designed to suggest possible directions for future research. In what follows, we argue that all outcome evaluations within nonprofit organizations present challenges to the evaluator/researcher and to the subject organizations, including the difficulty of specifying the appropriate outcome measures and resource constraints. Despite these common challenges, unique barriers exist for the evaluation of FBOs and secular programs.

In particular, this paper focuses on the following questions pertaining to the process of evaluating and comparing faith-based and secular organizations:

- What practical problems exist in conducting outcome or effectiveness evaluation of faith-based programs?
- What are the particular challenges that exist in comparing secular and faith-based organizations?
- What are the key issues of which researchers should be mindful for future research on faith based organizations?

DESCRIPTION OF THE COMPARATIVE STUDY

These case studies were conducted in three different service categories in three different parts of the country: (1) parent education in Mississippi (Bartkowski, 2004); (2) residential addiction programs in Washington and Oregon (Smith, 2004); and (3) transitional housing in Michigan (Grettenberger, 2004).

In each of the case studies, every effort was made to adhere to a similar protocol.[1] Briefly, this protocol involved the following steps. First, the universe of secular agencies and FBOs in one or more communities was identified for each separate case study. For example, all programs providing transitional housing services in a middle-sized city in Michigan were identified. A similar approach was employed in the other case study communities. Second, a minimum subset of agencies was selected from this universe of agencies for intensive study and examination. Ideally, agencies in the sample varied according to source of revenue and the role of faith in the agency. Consequently, this minimum subset of agencies included in each locale: one privately funded FBO; two publicly funded FBOs (with different levels of faith integration); and one publicly funded secular agency.

A central part of the comparative survey was the Faith Integration Survey (FIS). This survey was designed to determine the degree to which faith was integrated into program administration and service delivery of each agency in all of the policy domains. The FIS was designed as a filtering survey to be distributed to every service organization in the service category in a given community. Then, the subset of agencies to be studied intensively was to be selected from information obtained from the FIS survey results. In fact, preliminary information was obtained from the universe of agencies and then the FIS was administered to only the agencies selected for intensive study.

In the final selection of agencies for intensive study, adaptations of the basic protocol were undertaken in each case study in order to fit with the contours of the local service landscape and program availability. For example, there was often only one parenting program in a rural Mississippi community, thereby requiring the researcher to move beyond sampling all programs from a single locale; instead, programs were selected from locales that were geographically dispersed but situated in communities with similar characteristics. Moreover, where the three different research sites are considered, faith-based programs were more abundant in some locales than in others. Thus, the actual mix of agencies varied across the case studies, although each case study included several secular and faith-based agencies.

The next step in the research entailed conducting face-to-face qualitative interviews with key stakeholders. Agency and program staff persons were the first to be interviewed. Typically, the executive director was the point of entry into the organization, and basic survey data on the agency and program were collected prior to the administration of the qualitative interview instrument. Upon completing this interview with the executive director, interviews were conducted with the program directors and line staff. Then, focus groups with clients were conducted in each agency. Usually, the focus groups consisted of fewer than ten people and lasted less than an hour. All the interviews were conducted using a similar questionnaire.[3] A tailored questionnaire was employed with the different categories of interviewees.

CHALLENGES IN EVALUATING EFFECTIVENESS

A common evaluation challenge is the specification of the variable of interest. In the comparative study, definition of the variables and the categorization of organizations by faith content were accorded special attention. Indeed, these key steps proved to be difficult and complicated. While political discourse about the faith-based initiative somewhat blithely refers to faith-based and secular organizations as separate and easily distinguished entities, the experience of researchers in this study illustrates the inadequacy of such simplistic categorizations. Indeed, some faith-based agencies operated, by their own admission, primarily secular programs. And some secular programs encouraged religious practice and regarded themselves as deeply spiritual organizations. Thus, research conducted on this topic needs to be sensitive to the wide array of possible combinations between secular and faith-based characteristics at the organizational level and the program level, while also considering the prospect for faith to be explicitly manifested or implicitly present in organizations and programs.

Contemporary discourse often presumes that programmatic outcomes directly related to faith as a primary or contributing intervention can be identified and measured. Yet, the actual role of faith as part of a program intervention and the attendant outcomes are frequently poorly specified. Where parent education was concerned, faith-based parent educators would commonly tailor the curriculum–and, specifically, would modulate the faith content of the program–to meet the needs of clients. Thus, developing reliable definitions of what constitutes faith content as well as definitions of target outcomes is critical to developing reliable and valid research in this area. But recognizing the complexities of actual programming and the fact that exposure to faith may vary from one group of clients to the next, even in the same program, is also vital.

Outcomes Measures

Transformation is an especially important outcome construct in comparisons of secular and faith-based programs because a central assumption often advanced in the discourse on faith-based organizations is that a key difference between FBOs and secular organizations is the focus of FBOs on spiritual and emotional transformation. FBOs are regarded as "holistic" programs, offering love or unconditional regard and support as a part of the program intervention such as drug rehabilitation (Bush, 2004; see also Bartkowski & Regis, 2003; Wuthnow, 2004). One of the presumed outcomes of this holistic approach is transformation. Secular organizations are seen as being focused on objective measures of services, such as the number of persons served and amount of service delivered, partly in response to professional standards and the expectations of public and private funders (Sherman, 1995).

In general, scant literature exists defining transformation and its indicators. Indeed, Sherman (1995) acknowledges the difficulty of measuring transformation, but nonetheless suggests that holistic services focused on transformation can lead to a variety of behavioral and attitudinal changes including:

> changed language, faithful attendance in education/training program, increased punctuality and personal responsibility, willing-

ness to work, improved social relationship with staff, re-affiliation with family, avoidance of drugs, commitment to financial account-ability, greater reliability, and increasing initiative and enthusi-asm. (p. 5)

While also considering other more traditional outcomes, this study sought to determine whether transformation was among the outcomes of any of the programs studied. This goal proved to be difficult for many reasons. First, variation existed among service providers on the mean-ing and implications of transformation for clients and what program-matic aspects were linked to a transformative experience. Overall, the providers themselves struggled with understanding transformation (even the FBOs in the sample). In some cases, transformation was not an ex-plicit goal but was seen as an available option for those clients who desired it. For example, faith-based parent educators in Mississippi of-fered what the researcher called "spirituality a la carte," such that faith was among the menu of options available to clients. Thus, biblical verses were interwoven with practical tips for parenting so that the tastes of multiple audiences could be satisfied.

Among all of the service domains investigated, program staff did not generally use language such as "transformation." But often they ap-peared to reference planned or perceived changes in program partici-pants that went beyond the overt goals and objectives of the programs. For example, might it be classified as "transformation" if a person moved from being homeless to having a home, a steady job, and better parenting skills? What if the program was secular rather than faith-based? Was it transformation if a woman in a transitional housing pro-gram said that she had already believed God could help her, but that the caring of the staff at a faith-based transitional housing program helped her get back on her feet after a divorce? Has a substance abuse program client who states that his life had been changed by a higher power been transformed as a result of the program even if he is still using drugs? Many staff in substance abuse programs would argue that a person re-quires some type of transformation if he or she is to stop using drugs. However, such changes do not need to be manifested explicitly as reli-gious transformation. In short, the development of clearer, measurable definitions of transformation and other outcomes are needed.

Moreover, outcomes are more easily measured in some policy and programming domains than others. For example, successful outcomes for homeless clients in a transitional housing program may be under-stood rather straightforwardly as securing adequate long-term shelter.

However, parenting attitudes and skills are more difficult to measure, in part because they rely on subjective, self-reported measures and because parenting itself is composed of many different dimensions (e.g., discipline, attachment, support). Thus, outcome measures on research instruments should be designed with an appreciation for the level of complexity in the desired effects of program participation.

Classifying Faith-Based Organizations

The appropriate classification of the level of faith in organizations is another important challenge in conducting comparative research with faith-based and secular organizations. Unfortunately, classification of the amount of faith content and the intensity of the religious experience offered to participants was complex. The classification made in policy discussions about faith-based organizations is often quite simple: "either you are or are not" faith-based. Political definitions of what constitutes a faith-based organization includes perspectives such as "Any program emanating out of a church or a synagogue or a mosque is a faith-based program" (Bush, 2004) although as Wuthnow (2004) noted, such programs often contain less faith content than non-congregationally affiliated faith-based programs.

Researchers, however, have understood that faith-based organizations vary considerably in type, and in the quantity and quality of faith elements. Several efforts to develop classification approaches for the religious nature of organizations preceded this study (Monsma, 1996, 2004; Jeavons; 1997; Smith and Sosin, 2001; Sider and Unruh, 2004). Among the issues to consider in classification are the ways in which religion is manifested in a particular faith tradition and how that might be incorporated into interventions. One such approach, used in this study, was the Faith Integration Survey (FIS). It is designed to recognize both the amount of religious/faith content in the agency and the program, and to consider the organization's religious context in classifying a program.

All of the faith-based programs in this study were in the Christian tradition. The study's methodology recognized that faith, even for groups of Christian origin, cannot be categorized using a homogenous set of definitions. This methodological approach was helpful in distinguishing the extent to which organizations reflected, in practice, faith as it is defined within each of their faith traditions.

In practice, the FIS allows ordinal classification of the programs or organizations according to their degree of faith integration. Consequently, it offers the opportunity for the classification of the faith integration of the organizations. While valuable in sorting faith-based and secular organizations into different categories, the FIS instrument needs further use in the field in order to deepen our understanding of the implications for programmatic outcomes of differing levels of faith integration. In particular, further study and use of the FIS instrument would be helpful in discerning the specific connection between levels of faith integration and client outcomes.

Another challenge for researchers is the difficulty of comparing religious content across agencies. For instance, one agency might hold religious services but actual participation in the services may be voluntary. Another agency may have the same policy but because of the structure of the program, clients might feel obligated to participate. Further, this sense of obligation may vary from client to client or vary depending upon the staff on duty.

A related challenge is in the distinction between spiritual and religious experience or identification. In the comparative study, several secular agencies (including agencies that offered drug treatment, and parent education that was often coupled with child care) regarded their programs as deeply spiritual. Some of these agencies offered regular classes on spirituality as well as spiritual counseling by trained counselors or, in some cases, ministers. In other cases, references to spirituality were more indirect, and discussed in the context of employees' commitment to assisting clients or in motivating them to enter a "helping" field. But they did not regard their agencies as "faith-based" or religious, which they interpreted as adopting one specific faith and imposing it on clients and/or staff.

The FIS provides for differentiation between faith traditions. In the transitional housing case, four of the five programs were at least nominally faith-based organizations. The FIS allowed differential classification of each of the four faith-based organizations since different forms of faith expression were assessed by the instrument. For one organization, staff saw the way the staff cared about and prayed for the clients as evidence of faith. In another, the requirement that clients participate in weekly Bible study and attendance at a Christian worship service was an important expression of faith to the staff. Weighting the various measures of faith expression helps in the classification of religiosity, since it does not presume a single measure of religiosity. Further efforts are needed, however, to validate measures of different types of religious inputs and their effects on client outcomes. Does praying for clients at staff meetings lead to different outcomes than weekly Bible study? This level of complexity in classification of faith-based organizations has yet to be effectively achieved.

Implementation of Evaluation

Each step of the evaluation process presented challenges for implementation. Human subjects review slowed data collection considerably in some sectors, notably residential addiction services. In addition, samples of programs and clients were small in transitional housing programs (five programs, seven direct service staff, seventeen clients in focus groups). This problem reflects a more general research and policy problem. That is, many communities do not have extensive large numbers of organizations in a particular service category. Even sizable cities may have only a relative handful of homeless shelters or drug treatment agencies. Consequently, it is difficult for researchers to sample a sufficiently diverse mix of organizations to allow comparisons across various types of secular and faith-based agencies.

The small sample size in turn posed challenges for interpreting and generalizing findings. Selection of programs and clients were not randomized. Client attrition from programs, with no follow-up on the part of the programs, further limited sampling for the study. Client attrition, of course, can promote a "creaming" effect for the program, such that a select group of participants are most likely to complete the program. However, the extent of creaming was not discernible. Tracking clients post-intervention presented similar problems for program staff. For example, most drug treatment agencies and parent education programs do not have the resources to track clients post-treatment. Thus, outcomes measures tended to be more process-related (such as attrition rates).

In general, our comparative study strongly indicated the need to address the complexity and differences of various programs when conducting cross-sector studies, due to important program-specific evaluation issues. Each of these issues will be discussed in detail below, with examples and illustrations from cases in this study.

Human Subjects Review

The process of project approval from university human subjects review committees is a necessary if sometimes slow process. It is relatively predictable experience, however, and one that can normally be negotiated. However, human subjects review is also a basically linear process whereupon each step in obtaining the required consent from agency staff and clients is envisioned as building upon the previous one. However, we found with small agencies, especially in the addiction field, that agency directors would not give consent until they had actually met with the researcher and learned more about the research process.

Larger, multi-site service agencies also present additional complications. First, many executives of larger agencies are essentially unavailable for in-depth interviews and they tend to know very little about the details of some of the specific programs (so they were not in a position, for example, to comment on the operations of the residential addiction programs). Second, larger agencies especially hospital or medical facilities usually have their own human subjects review process. Thus, even with university human subject review approval, the researchers were required to undergo another round of review at these agencies. In some cases, the review was so complicated and lengthy that the agency was dropped from the study.

Sample Size

Securing adequate sample size was another sector-specific barrier. In transitional housing, for example, only six prospective programs existed that met the parameters established by the FIS protocol. All but one of these programs was quite small. Consequently, the number of programs available to participate and the number of staff available for the interviews was quite limited. The client focus groups were also quite small (as was also the case with parent education focus groups). More specifically, even though all current staff and most current clients participated in the study for the four small programs, each sample was very small. Four of the five transitional housing programs had only one direct service worker. And while the numbers of active clients varied, three programs housed no more than three families at a time. Additionally, the length of programs (approximately two years) made it difficult to secure former participants for interviews. (Tracking former participants is also discussed in a later section.) As a result, the researchers needed to be very cautious about the reliability and generalizability of the data collected.

The size of organizations is particularly relevant to the comparative study of FBOs and secular organizations. One argument for a greater role of FBOs in providing social services is that they are more community grounded and responsive, in part because they are viewed as smaller and less bureaucratic. The programs in this study did not necessarily support either assumption, as several of the programs identified as faith-based were embedded in organizations that were considerably larger than their secular counterparts. Size was not a function of faith connection. Indeed, many of the programs in the study, both secular and faith-based, were small. Leaving aside the question of whether FBOs are more community grounded and less bureaucratic, it is clear that there are many small programs, at least in some sectors. The small size of many of these organizations also means that the agency characteristics reflect the religious beliefs of the individual staff members rather than a coherent approach to faith content in services. In short, small organizational size is an ongoing challenge for any research in this area.

Self-Selection of Programs

Minimally, full participation by either a representative sample of the universe of existing programs within the target areas would have provided the best research methodology. But the practical difficulties encountered in the real world of service agencies prevented the study researchers from achieving this goal. For instance, some programs chose not to participate in the study but they represented a wide variety of different types of agencies. While it is difficult to discern the specific reasons for the refusal of some organizations to participate, it is quite possible that programs with a reputation for poor quality services were less inclined to participate. Also, programs lodged within larger facilities with their own review process were also less likely to participate (largely due to the staff time involved in obtaining approval from their superiors).

Further, many faith-intensive programs were even eager to participate. For example, some faith-based parenting programs regarded the interviews with researchers as an opportunity to broadcast their faith message, get additional exposure for their program, and discuss their accomplishments (e.g., lives changed, networks established). This strong desire to participate in the research project was also evident among drug treatment agencies. This is not to suggest that self-serving reasons were behind the participation of these programs in the study. However, this pattern does underscore that potential for some programs to use all available resources–including their participation in a research study–to spread their message and alert policymakers and potential clients to their program.

This pattern was not evident in the transitional housing case, where six programs were identified by the researchers as meeting the criteria for the study. Five programs, spread across the continuum of faith content, agreed to participate. However one program, which is widely known in the community as having the most religious content and mandatory participation, declined to participate (without knowing much about the study).

Staff and Self-Selection of Clients

For many reasons, a random or representative sample of clients was infeasible. The involvement of staff in identifying prospective participants in the study acted as a filter for the clients selected to participate or asked to volunteer. Also, the staff's level of cooperation influenced the amount of effort put into recruiting clients for the focus groups. For instance, in one transitional housing program, staff members were reluctant to recruit clients other that the two parents who were currently housed.

The self-selection of clients for the focus groups varied depending by service category. In transitional housing, clients were able to opt out of participation. It is not unreasonable to assume that persons who were most involved in the programs were also most likely to be seen as appropriate for participation by staff and most likely to be agree to cooperate with that selection. It is also likely that successful participants were more likely to attend the focus group as scheduled. This selection process would most logically be biased toward more successful program participants.

In addiction programs, less formal screening was done by program staff, partly due to the nature of the programs. Typically, the staff simply announced that the researcher was available for a focus group with interested participants. In some of the larger programs, the clients who chose to participate tended to be individuals with a special interest in religion or spirituality. In smaller programs, the clients in the focus groups represented a wide variety of perspectives including many unmotivated clients and clients with no particular interest in religion or spirituality.

In parent education programs, it was difficult to enlist clients in the study. Most of the faith-based programs in this study were fatherhood programs. It was explained to the researcher that program clients were initially wary of participating in the program (and hence any evaluation of it) because they feared that the government would impose child support payments on them. Also, funding for the fatherhood programs ended just as the client focus group phase of the study was getting underway. Thus, interviews were conducted in focus groups for some programs and one-on-one in others.

Client Attrition

Proper measurement of outcomes should include all persons who have participated in programs. Client attrition from programs confounds the ability of researchers to sample from all persons who have been influenced by a program intervention. However, programs were unable to locate program drop-outs. Many did not reliably track participants who dropped out of the programs, even at a basic level of keeping track of the numbers.

The smaller transitional housing programs sometimes were able to estimate the number of dropouts because they could essentially identify them. The staff of the larger programs were not even sure how many or what percentage of participants dropped out, although there may have been a record from which that could have been calculated. In addiction programs, client attrition is even a debatable measure and most programs (especially the smaller programs or the programs that did not rely on government funding) did not carefully track attrition rates. In parent education, completion of the program was much more likely among those who were court-mandated to take the course or risk having their children removed from their home because of child abuse or neglect. Women were more commonly court-mandated, thus creating a lack of gender parity in program utilization and completion.

Tracking Clients Post-Intervention

Ideally, outcomes would also be measured by tracking the clients who successfully completed the entire program. For example, if a drug treatment program is designed for six months, the outcomes would be measured by learning the status of clients six months or a year after the completion of the program. For the purposes of this study, having more program graduates would have resulted in better data, and that was the intended design. Focus groups were to have included a combination of program graduates and current participants. This proved to be nearly impossible in many instances, with program staff readily acknowledging their inability to track program participants following their receipt of services. The problem of tracking clients reflected in part the resource difficulties. But it also reflected problems in locating clients who often have very transient lifestyles.

To be sure, many programs try to obtain information on ex-participants in their programs. For instance, many agencies offering transitional housing, residential addiction treatment, and parent education are often visited by former clients who sometimes stop by to say "hello." Some programs (namely, addiction and parent education) tried to learn more about ex-clients by organizing "alumni" get-togethers. These events offered an opportunity to obtain information and provide some modicum of social support. In general, it seems reasonable to assume that these reunions tend to attract the more successful former participants.

Controlling for the Faith Factor

One challenge in controlling for the faith factor is that clients may often receive multiple services, either simultaneously or over a period of months or years. For persons with substance abuse problems, it is common for individuals to have multiple treatment episodes. This is true for homeless services as well. In addition, it is common for homeless persons to transition from one program type (such as emergency shelter) to another (such as transitional housing). In fact, one HUD criteria that may be used to qualify a homeless person to receive transitional housing services is to be coming from an emergency shelter. As a result, homeless persons may receive services from multiple sources, including both faith-based and secular organizations. In parent education programs, parent education is often "bundled" with other services such as GED completion or employment referrals. The essential point is that programs often exhibit complexity in service delivery that makes isolating the faith factor quite difficult.

SUGGESTIONS FOR FUTURE RESEARCH

The findings of our study suggest three key areas that need attention in future research projects on faith-based organizations: (1) the classification of religious or spiritual levels and content of programs (including programs identified as secular); (2) the specification of outcome variables; and (3) client attrition.

Classification of the concept "faith-based" is essential in conducting comparative research with secular and faith-based organizations. However, a basic continuum of religiosity is inadequate for the purposes of comparing program outcomes. The FIS used in this study provides an important and valuable tool in conceptualizing and measuring the faith content of the service programs. Further validation and refinement of the FIS would be helpful, particularly in establishing how faith is expressed within the tradition with which the program is affiliated.

Two steps seem most important in specifying the variables for outcome measurement. One is to clarify whose definitions of outcomes are to be used, and to be quite careful in the way that outcomes are treated. In current evaluation parlance, outcomes are defined quite narrowly and are considered the holy grail of program performance. However, studying outcomes as "effects" of program participation without an appreciation for the more complex processes behind them can be fraught with peril. For example, instructors and participants in parent education programs often discussed the consciousness-raising that occurred during the course of such programs. Participants who thought they were good parents upon entry into the program learned that there was a lot they did not know about parenting during the program. As explained by one parent educator, if the same self-evaluation of parenting was administered at intake and upon program completion, the program completion score was often not greater than the intake score, and sometimes was even lower. In such circumstances, the parents' attention to the details of child-rearing (e.g., how often do I praise my child?) had been sharpened, resulting in a lower and more accurate score on such an item.

Improving client retention in the evaluation process is an important step toward more effective evaluation. Developing effective means of finding clients who have discontinued services are also needed. Yet, assessing reasons why clients drop out of programs is also relevant. On this important dimension, client attrition of FBO and secular programs should be investigated. Some programs may have different success rates. Further, more information is needed on the reasons for client attrition from various programs including whether or not the faith elements or programs have any bearing on retention in programs. This type of evaluation would require planning and flexibility on the part of the programs and researchers.

In sum, this study is part of a growing body of literature on the characteristics of faith-based and secular organizations (Chaves, 2004; Monsma, 2004; Wuthnow, 2004). Yet, a lot of research remains to be conducted, especially with regard to comparing the outcomes of faith-based and secular organizations. One enduring lesson of this study is that research can be very valuable in building the knowledge base and helping identify key issues for further study. But the very characteristics of many secular and faith-based social service agencies that make them attractive to policymakers and citizens, such as their small size and relative informality, pose evaluation challenges that make a definitive judgment on the relative effectiveness and efficiency of these agencies quite elusive.

NOTES

1. This paper is based on research that was supported by the Rockefeller Institute at the State University of New York (SUNY) at Albany and the Pew Charitable Trust. Special thanks are extended to Richard Nathan and David Wright of the Rockefeller Institute for their support and feedback. Also see, Bartkowski, 2004; Grettenberger, 2004; Smith, 2004; and Smith, Bartowski, and Grettenberger, 2004.

2. See Goggin and Orth, 2002.

3. This questionnaire was developed by the Rockefeller Institute.

REFERENCES

Bartkowski, J.P. (2004). Faith-based and secular parenting programs in rural Mississippi: A comparative case study. Manuscript submitted for publication.

Bartkowski, J.P., and Regis, H.A. (2003). *Charitable Choices: Religion, Race, and Poverty in the Post-Welfare Era*. New York: New York University Press.

Bush, G.W. (2001). Rallying the armies of compassion. Retrieved on March 1, 2001 from http://www.whitehouse.gov/news/reports/faithbased.html

Bush, G.W. (2004). Remarks by the President to faith-based and community leaders. Union Bethel AME Church. New Orleans, LA. Retrieved on January 20, 2004 from http://www.whitehouse.gov/news/releases/2004/01/print/20040115-7.html

Bush, G.W. (March,2005). President highlights faith-based initiative at Leadership Conference. Retrieved on April 2, 2005 from http://www.whitehouse.gove/news/releases/200503/print/200503014.html

Carlson-Theis, S. (2004). "Implementing the faith-based initiative," *The Public Interest,* Sp (155), 57-74.

Chaves, M. (2004). *Congregations in America*. Harvard University Press: Cambridge, MA.

DiIulio, J.J. (2004). Getting faith-based programs right. *The Public Interest*, Sp (155), 75-88.

Goggin, M.L., & Orth, D. (2002). *How faith-based and secular organizations tackle housing for the homeless*. Albany, N.Y: Rockefeller Institute.

Grettenberger, S. (2004). Transitional housing in a midwest community: A comparative study of faith-based and secular programs. Paper presented at the 33rd Annual Conference of Association for Research on Nonprofit Organizations and Voluntary Action. Los Angeles.

Herman, R.D., & Renz, D.O. (n.d.). *Nonprofit organizational effectiveness: Practical implications of research on an elusive concept*. Midwest Center for Nonprofit Leadership: Kansas City, MO.

Jeavons, T. (1997). Identifying characteristics of "religious" organizations: An exploratory proposal. In J. Demerath III, P.D. Hall, T. Schmitt, & R.H. Williams (Eds.). *Sacred companies: Organizational aspects of religion and religious aspect of organizations* (pp. 79-95). New York: Oxford University Press.

Mecca, W.F., Rivera, A., & Esposito, A.J. (2000). Instituting an outcomes assessment effort: Lessons from the field. Families in Society, 81(1), 85-89.

Monsma, S.V. (1996). *When sacred and secular mix: Religious nonprofit organizations and public money.* Lanham, MD: Rowman & Littlefield.

Monsma, S.V. (2004). *Putting Faith in Partnerships: Welfare to Work in Four Cities.* Ann Arbor: University of Michigan Press.

Monsma, S.V., & Mounts, C.M. (2002). *Working faith: How religious organizations provide welfare-to-work services.* Center for Research on Religion and Urban Civil Society.

Morley, E., Vinson, E., & Hatry, H.P. (2001). *Outcome measurement in nonprofit organizations: Current practices and recommendations.* Washington, DC: Independent Sector.

Mulroy, E.A., & Lauber, H. (2004). A user-friendly approach to program evaluation and effective community interventions for families at risk of homelessness. *Social Work*, 49, 573-586.

Ragan, M. (2004). *Faith-based vs. secular: Using administrative data to compare the performance of faith-affiliated and other social service providers.* Rockefeller Institute of Government: Albany, NY.

Rock, J. (2002). *Stepping out on faith: New York City's charitable choice demonstration program.* Rockefeller Institute of Government: Albany, NY.

Sherman, A.L. (1995). "Cross purposes," *Policy Review.* 74(Fall), 58-63.

Sider, R.J., & Unruh, H.R. (2004). Typology of religious characteristics of social service and educational organization and programs. *Nonprofit and Voluntary Sector Quarterly*, 33, 109-134.

Smith, S.R. (2004). Faith-based and secular drug and alcohol treatment programs In Washington and Oregon: A comparative case study. Paper presented at the 33rd Annual Conference of Association for Research on Nonprofit Organizations and Voluntary Action. Los Angeles.

Smith, S.R., Bartkowski, J., & Grettenberger, S. (2004). Comparative Case Studies of Faith-Based And Secular Service Agencies: An Overview. Albany, NY: Reckefeller Institute, SUNY-Albany.

Smith, S.R., & Sosin, M.R. (2001). The varieties of faith-related agencies. *Public Administration Review,* 61(6): 651-670.

Somers, C.L., & Piliawsky, M. (2004). Drop-out prevention among urban, African American adolescents: Program evaluation and practical implications. *Preventing School Failure*, 48(3), 17-22.

Soskis, B. (2001). What religion cannot do: Act of faith. *The New Republic.* 224(9), 20-13.

Whipple, E.E., & Nathans, L.L. (2005) Evaluation of a rural Health Families America (HFA) program: The Importance of context. *Families in Society*, 86(1), 71-82.

Wuthnow, R. (2004). *Saving America? Faith-based services and the future of civil society.* Princeton University Press: Princeton.

Chapter 12

Assessing the Effectiveness of Faith-Based Programs: A Local Network Perspective

David Campbell
Eric Glunt

SUMMARY. The policy debate over faith-based initiatives has prompted calls for comparative effectiveness research. Drawing examples from an evaluation of California's Community and Faith-based Initiative (CFBI), we illustrate a research strategy that takes local networks as the primary unit of analysis. This approach focuses on understanding the roles different organizations play within local service delivery networks, and on analyzing how local actors coordinate services to affect participant, organization, and system outcomes. The network perspective casts new light on policy options, and suggests that caution is necessary when using administrative data to interpret program effectiveness.

David Campbell, PhD, is Community Studies Specialist, Department of Human and Community Development, 1 Shields Avenue, University of California, Davis, CA 95616 (E-mail: dave.c.campbell@ucdavis.edu). Eric Glunt, PhD, is Assistant Professor, Department of Occupational Studies, California State University, Long Beach.

[Haworth co-indexing entry note]: "Assessing the Effectiveness of Faith-Based Programs: A Local Network Perspective." Campbell, David, and Eric Glunt. Co-published simultaneously in *Journal of Religion & Spirituality in Social Work* (The Haworth Pastoral Press, an imprint of The Haworth Press, Inc.) Vol. 25, No. 3/4, 2006, pp. 241-259; and: *Faith-Based Social Services: Measures, Assessments, and Effectiveness* (ed: Stephanie C. Boddie, and Ram A. Cnaan) The Haworth Pastoral Press, an imprint of The Haworth Press, Inc., 2006, pp. 241-259.

KEYWORDS. Faith-based organizations, outcome effectiveness, networks, local service delivery

One of the few points of agreement in the debate over "faith-based" or "charitable choice" policy initiatives is that little rigorous evidence exists to document the efficacy of faith-based programs (Burke, Fossett, & Gais, 2004; Johnson, 2002; Monsma, 2002; Ragan, 2004; Smith & Sosin, 2001). In this context "rigorous" is often equated with research designs that take individual programs as the unit of analysis, assume that clients participate in only one type of program, and then compare outcomes across programs using standard, single metric indicators, such as job placement rates (Deb & Jones, 2003; Ragan, 2004). The question posed is whether faith-based or secular programs are more cost-effective, using available indicators of cost and outcomes.

Without denigrating this approach, we want to suggest an alternative research strategy that takes seriously the context in which individual programs operate, and seeks to rigorously describe and understand the complexities of how services are actually organized and delivered at the local level. In this approach the unit of analysis is the local service delivery network, comprised of public agencies and a variety of faith-related and secular nonprofit organizations. A fundamental assumption is that program participants are served by multiple agencies, often sequentially and sometimes simultaneously. Viewed from the perspective of a single local organization, Figure 1 provides a simplified picture of the diverse entities that constitute a local workforce delivery network, and highlights how any single entity is part of a complex inter-organizational field.

As we hope to demonstrate, careful process evaluations that take network dynamics seriously are important for two reasons. First, they can inform the analysis of administrative data and guard against faulty interpretations. Second, they can bring into view a broader array of effectiveness questions, based on the outcomes that influence local implementation. From the participant perspective, what matters is not so much the quality of any particular service they receive but how the overall service portfolio they assemble by contacting different community organizations aids or hinders their progress. From the organizational perspective, the question is whether existing roles and the accompanying patterns of conflict and cooperation with the network strengthen or undermine organizational capacity and resilience. From the system perspective, the question is how effectively network actors are cooperating to achieve

FIGURE 1. Local Network Relationships of CFBOs Involved in Workforce Development

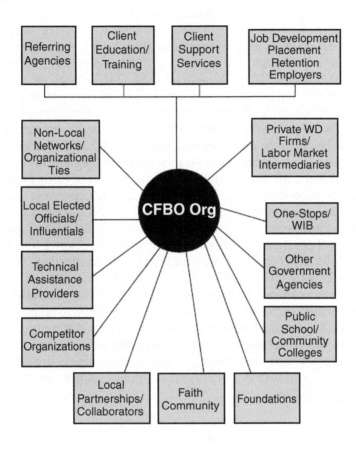

results of public value (Moore, 1995; Renz & Herman, 2004; Wuthnow, 2004).

To illustrate methods and insights associated with the local network perspective, we draw on data from a 3-year evaluation of the California Community and Faith-based Initiative (CFBI).[1] Through a competitive grant process managed by the California Employment Development Department (EDD), CFBI funded 30 faith-based and 10 secular non-profit organizations to help hard-to-employ individuals prepare for, find, and retain employment.[2] Using more than $17 million in state and federal funds, CFBI served more than 6,000 program participants including the homeless, ex-offenders, recovering substance abusers, emancipated foster care youth, autistic youth, abused women, mental health clients, and refugees and new immigrants. As designed under the administration of Governor Gray Davis and approved by the state legislature, CFBI grantees included many smaller and less established nonprofit organizations that had never previously received government grants. The primary CFBI goals were twofold: (1) to expand the reach of workforce development services to individuals not served by traditional government programs, and (2) to build the capacity of community-based organizations to operate effectively and accountably as government partners. At the height of the program, more than 20 EDD staff were assigned to provide extensive technical assistance to funded organizations.[3]

As researchers, we were initially drawn to the idea of using the CFBI evaluation to produce conventional comparative effectiveness data using individual programs as the level of analysis. But the deeper we inquired into CFBI goals, the practices of funded organizations, and the experiences of program participants, the more we were drawn into viewing the California initiative from a local network perspective. The following pages provide a condensed account of the evolution of our thinking as it was shaped by accumulating findings from the evaluation. As we eventually discovered, a local network perspective helps illuminate useful distinctions between the roles played by different types of community and faith-based organizations (CFBOs) in relation to other network actors. We discuss how these distinctions might inform the interpretation of administrative data and the policy choices surrounding faith-based initiatives.

LITERATURE REVIEW

Charitable choice provisions in the 1996 welfare reform legislation sought to expand partnerships between faith-based organizations and government. A 2002 Hudson Institute study (Green & Sherman, 2002) found that the number of such partnerships had indeed grown and that more than half of the faith-based organizations involved were new to government contracting. Summarizing the early experience, Sherman (2002, p. 99) states:

> . . . it is very possible for the faith community to make an ever-larger contribution to meeting America's social needs but highly

improbable that it can replace government's role completely. Discernment is needed to identify the unique strengths and capacities of the faith sector–and the unique strengths and capacities of the public sector–and to devise strategies that draw upon the distinctive characteristics and special resources of each.

Since 2002, the Compassion Capital Fund of the Bush administration has earmarked funding to intermediary organizations that provide technical assistance and sub-awards to local faith-based organizations. A similar initiative within the Department of Labor funds intermediaries with the specific goal of increasing collaboration between government-supported One-Stop Career Centers and the faith community, an explicit recognition of the need for a partnership between public workforce development programs and community and faith-based organizations. The state of California initiative discussed here sought to develop such a partnership. Rather than fund an external intermediary, California chose to use the special projects unit within the Employment Development Department as the local capacity building agent.

Community and faith-based organizations with deep community connections have the potential to expand the reach of social services and serve as portals into public programs. Evaluations of government job training programs consistently find that service providers avoid enrolling hard-to-employ participants in order to meet performance standards more readily (Franklin & Ripley, 1984; Magnum, 2000). The Workforce Investment Act of 1998 (WIA) exacerbates this disincentive by eliminating the past practice of adjusting local performance measures to take into account client characteristics and local economic circumstances (Brustein & Knight, 1998). WIA also stipulates that employers are primary customers of the system of One-Stop career centers that serve local areas. One-Stop operators, who must meet high performance standards and gain the confidence of employers, find it difficult to reach out to individuals with multiple barriers to employment. CFBI was conceived in part with the goal of filling the resulting service delivery gap, and tested the idea that it is more cost-effective to do so by using nonprofit CFBOs who are adept at working with particular geographic, cultural, or linguistic populations.

To assess CFBI success, our evaluation was initially designed to document the reach and effectiveness of One-Stop and CFBI programs. The literature suggested two relevant hypotheses about the likely effectiveness of different types of organizations serving hard-to-employ individuals. The hypothesis undergirding faith-based policy initiatives is that the commitments, culture, and resources of faith-related organizations have a unique potential to change lives (Cisneros, 1996; Cnaan, Wineburg, & Boodie, 2000; Glenn, 2000; Monsma, 1996). Specific features of faith-related organizations hypothesized to contribute to their success include community connections and legitimacy, holistic and highly personal attention to the material and spiritual needs of clients, attention to changing inner attitudes and motivations, a more inviting and less bureaucratic organizational culture, and–more controversially–the incorporation of specific religious practices (e.g., prayer, Bible study) into programs.

A competing hypothesis is that larger and more established employment and training organizations (whether faith-related or not) with professional staffs and extensive community networks are better equipped to work with hard-to-employ populations (Kramer, Nightingale et al., 2002; Smith & Sosin, 2001). For example, one study finds that workforce development organizations with frequent, close, and long-term contact with employers are better at placing individuals in jobs (Harrison & Weiss, 1998).

FIELD RESEARCH ACTIVITIES AND FINDINGS

Initial Survey of Organizations

With these considerations in mind, we conducted an initial survey of CFBI organizations that asked questions about their organization and programs. The responses suggested the possibility of developing effectiveness comparisons using a matrix (see Table 1) based on two variables: the strength of the faith connection (high-to-moderate vs. low-to-none) and the longevity of the sponsoring organization (more established vs. newer).[4] The original research design called for in-depth case studies of at least 3-4 organizations from each of the four cells, and for comparing reach and outcome data across the four cells using administrative data gathered by EDD from all 40 organizations.

Even as we created this design, however, two findings from the same survey began to raise troubling questions about the validity of the comparisons it sought. First, faith-based practices played a relatively small role in the services provided by CFBOs. Of the 28 respondents we interviewed from faith-based organizations (the other 10 being from secular organizations), more than two-thirds indicated that faith was the motivating factor in why they did the work (N = 21), or a source of tangible

TABLE 1. Initial Design to Compare Effectiveness

Organizational Longevity	Strength of Faith Connection	
	High-to-Moderate	Low-to-None
Newer	11	9
More established	8	10

Numbers in cells represent the total cases in the sample, based on initial analysis of 38 scoping surveys. Two organizations did not participate in the survey.

resources that supported the work (N = 25).[5] But only 4 of the 28 indicated that they used faith-based practices, such as prayer or Bible reading, in their activities with program participants. All of these were careful to note that such activities were voluntary. While not surprising (EDD had made it a point to educate funded organizations that required sectarian activities were not permitted), this finding immediately raised the issue of whether any observed differences in the outcomes of faith-related organizations could be meaningfully linked to their faith-orientation or practices. For example, is a job training program with an essentially secular orientation conceptually distinct simply because it is run by a faith-related organization? If so, how would it be distinguished from a similar public agency program run by staff who happened to be people of faith?

Second, many CFBOs indicated that workforce development activities were secondary to their primary organizational mission, such as promoting sober living, providing transitional housing, or offering counseling services. Only 11 of the 38 organizations reported extensive prior experience with workforce programs, and 16 had no experience. In many cases, the organization's workforce development efforts were a relatively minor part of their overall interaction with clients.

While all the organizations saw a connection between workforce development activities and their primary goals, it would be unfair to judge their effectiveness using job placement and retention outcomes as the sole measures. Program staff consistently said that they measured success in small steps and in areas that administrative data do not capture, such as "whether a participant calls us when they can't make an appointment," or whether they "keep coming back" even when a job is not immediately forthcoming. The outcomes that mattered to these organizations were expressed in terms such as "giving clients hope," "building self-esteem," and "creating a sense of family." While it was clear that these outcomes make an important difference in the lives of participants, it was apparent that they would be difficult or impossible to correlate with immediate gains in employment.

Field Interviews with Program Staff and Participants

We used interviews with program staff and with randomly selected program participants to explore how the services provided by CFBOs fit into the overall mix of agencies with which participants interacted, both prior to and during the grant period. Two findings were of particular note. First, of the more than 150 participants interviewed, 42% indicated that they had never previously received workforce development services. Reasons included lack of a car or access to transportation, distance lived from the nearest One-Stop, being suspicious or fearful of government, or language barriers. Second, program participants typically had contact with multiple community agencies. For example, more than 36% of interviewees reported that their CFBI program had referred them to another community agency service, and 40% had come to the CFBI program after being referred by a public agency, including those who were court-referred. This evidence calls into question a key presumption in conventional comparative effectiveness research–the idea that client outcomes are the product of a single organization and its program. Indeed, by the third year of CFBI, EDD program managers expected each CFBO to have developed a relationship with a local One-Stop as part of their required performance benchmarks.

Network Mapping and Analysis

At about the mid-way point of our 3-year evaluation, we launched a second phase of research focused specifically on understanding the roles and relationships of CFBOs within local networks, including their One-Stop connections. We studied 14 organizations in 11 different local workforce investment areas. The analysis used a variety of methods, including the construction of a network map showing the connections of each CFBO to employers, funders, government agencies, technical assistance providers, other faith-related organizations, community coalitions and partnerships, social and political leaders, and competitor organizations (see Figure 1). This exercise illustrated the complexity of workforce development networks, and the wide range of relationships which leaders of CFBOs must manage. To learn more about these relationships, and about how the CFBOs are valued as partners, we conducted 14 interviews with leaders of the participating CFBOs, 48 with representatives of One-Stop centers, local Workforce Investment Boards, and other government agencies, and 25 with employers and CBO partners. This community network analysis revealed three distinct roles played by CFBOs in local workforce networks:

1. a source of *remedial care and services* that offers an alternative portal into the workforce development system;
2. the developer of an *alternative employment and training network* that connects hard-to-employ participants with services and jobs tailored to their unique culture, language, and/or situations; and
3. the provider of a *specialized service* to which One-Stops (or other agencies) can refer participants when they are ready.

Depending on which of the three roles they play, CFBOs have different strengths and limitations as service providers and as One-Stop partners. Organizations emphasizing *remedial care* helped participants achieve basic outcomes that constitute the lower rungs of the self-sufficiency ladder: gaining trust, sobriety, emotional support, social skills, and self-confidence. The six remedial care organizations we studied feature low staff-participant ratios (averaging 1 to 8), close relationships between staff and participants (rather than bureaucratic encounters, see Gutek, 1995), and program designs that encourage peer support. Successful graduates of remedial care programs are ready to use employment and training services at One-Stops or other facilities.

Organizations emphasizing the *alternative network* role become a full-service alternative whose services that run parallel to those of One-Stops, but excel at reaching into particular geographic or cultural communities. Unlike remedial care organizations, these organizations ensure that participants have access to more advanced job training and job placement services, either by developing them as part of their own service portfolio or by establishing collaborative connections to other providers. For example, many CFBOs in this category seek out employers who are willing to take a chance on individuals with criminal records, drug involvement, or checkered work histories. Not surprisingly, the five organizations in this category averaged more than four times as many organizational connections as those in the remedial services category. Three of the five alternative network organizations we studied had created an active partnership with a nearby One-Stop that went beyond simple referrals. Compared to the smaller and younger remedial care organizations, all five alternative network organizations had been in existence for at least 8 years and had relatively large budgets and staff.

Three of our 14 organizations offered a *specialized service* to which existing participants in One-Stops or other public and nonprofit agencies can be referred. These CFBOs tend to serve relatively higher numbers of participants, but in a more limited fashion than in the other cases.

A NETWORK PERSPECTIVE ON EFFECTIVENESS

The network role distinctions we identified turned out to play a critical role in how we interpreted effectiveness data gathered in the course of our evaluation. Taking seriously the notion that "nonprofit effectiveness is a social construction" (Renz & Herman, 2004), we asked state and local workforce development officials to assess the contributions of EDD-funded CFBOs. We also conducted a preliminary analysis of administrative data provided by EDD regarding the demographic characteristics and employment outcomes of CFBI participants. In each case, a network perspective adds crucial insight.

Perspectives of State and Local Workforce Officials

In a notable departure from its typical practices, EDD devoted considerable time and resources to helping CFBOs develop their organizational policies and procedures, accounting capacity, grant writing expertise, and other components of organizational capacity. EDD staff we interviewed revealed that these activities were particularly time consuming with the smaller, less-established community organizations that specialized in providing remedial care. Clear tradeoffs came to light. While a few program managers suggested that it was not cost-effective to fund organizations in existence less than a year or two, others insisted that the newer organizations brought fresh ideas and passion and often were the only ones to serve the neediest populations locally.

In an attempt to codify the program managers' assessments, we gave them a series of statements that asked them to rate the overall promise of the 40 funded CFBOs as government partners. Using a Likert scale, program managers agreed or strongly agreed that 31 of the 40 organizations were effective overall partners. This group included 10 of the 19 organizations that had been in existence for six years or less. Newer organizations emphasizing remedial care are overrepresented among the nine rated as less effective. Three of the 4 organizations identified as deficient partners had been in existence three years or less, and 4 of the 5 who were given a "neutral" or "not sure" rating had been in existence for six years or less.

Interview data from local One-Stop and Workforce Investment Board officials fit a clear pattern: local leaders are skeptical about faith-based initiatives in the abstract and critical of the decision by Governor Davis to use WIA discretionary funds for CFBI, but speak in consistently positive terms about the contributions of particular CFBI-funded organizations in their own communities. One WIB director's comments capture the dichotomy:

> Some of the CFBI money came here, and we partnered with those organizations that got funded in our area. We were lucky. It works with those that got funded in our area. But from the time I was a child we were taught about the separation of church and state. These organizations do some good work, but they can't begin to comply, the small ones anyway, not the large ones. They don't have the capability and they don't have the accountability.

One reason CFBI was viewed negatively is because it allocated the governor's WIA 15% discretionary funds to nonprofit programs at a time when budget cuts were hampering the ability of the One-Stop system to maintain its basic infrastructure. Local officials also did not like the fact that they were not consulted on which organizations were selected, and believe it is unwise to provide government funds to groups with minimal or no track record.

Running somewhat counter to the call for rigorous side-by-side comparisons of faith-based and secular programs, local network officials appeared to base their specific effectiveness judgments on whether local CFBOs fill an important niche and on their longer-term promise as partners. By far the most consistent criticisms we heard from local officials did not focus on the issues of nonprofit capacity or quality. Instead, they feared the lack of stable, long-term funding associated with a state initiative, raising the prospect that efforts spent developing organizational partnerships would be too short-lived to be worthwhile.

Interpreting Administrative Data

As EDD program managers reminded the funded organizations, unless they could provide evidence that their programs were meeting WIA performance standards for job placement and retention, it would be hard for the organizations to attract future funding after CFBI ended.[6] But what if administrative data tells a misleading story?

Our analysis of CFBI administrative data is still underway. We have complete demographic information on the types of individuals CFBOs have served, but only 55% of all participants (3,387 out of 6,136) have been officially measured for outcomes due to time lags in data reporting. The results to date reveal interesting patterns that bear further investigation. For starters, CFBOs have served significantly higher percentages of the hard-to-employ in each of seven categories (see Table 2). By partnering with CFBOs, California significantly extended the reach of its workforce services to the disadvantaged. For example, CFBI funding led to a 74% increase in the number of homeless individuals in California who received WIA-funded workforce development services, and a 56% increase among those who self-declare as having issues with substance abuse.

A comparison of the job placement rates at exit for all WIA adult participants in California One-Stop programs against those for all CFBI participants for whom data are currently available shows CFBOs lagging far behind (70% to 40%; see Table 3). In an attempt to control for

TABLE 2. Percentage of One-Stop and CFBI Participants in Seven Hard-to-Employ Categories

% of All Served (Count)	WIA Formula Adults (N = 46,897)	All CFBI Adults (N = 6,136)	% Increase in Number Served in California	Remedial Care CFBI adults (N = 1,728)	Alternative Network CFBI Adults (N = 1,513)	Specialized Services CFBI Adults (N = 1,179)
Homeless	4.2% (1,978)	23.8% (1,461)	+ 74%	24.7% (426)	21.0% (317)	11.3% (133)
Substance Abuse	4.9% (2,302)	21.0% (1,291)	+ 56%	31.9% (552)	25.8% (391)	5.1% (60)
Disability	6.3% (2,979)	15.3% (941)	+ 32%	23.5% (407)	8.5% (129)	9.4% (111)
Ex-Offenders	14.3% (6,724)	27.7% (1,703)	+ 25%	36.4% (629)	32.8% (497)	5.5% (65)
On Public Assistance	24.7% (11,567)	47.6% (2,923)	+ 25%	54.2% (936)	36.7% (556)	60.7% (716)
Less than High School Degree	16.8% (7,872)	20.2% (1,238)	+ 16%	27.8% (480)	24.3% (367)	9.2% (109)
Low-Income	68.5% (32,136)	85.8% (5,265)	+ 16%	89.2% (1,542)	87.4% (1,322)	83.0% (978)

Source: California Employment Development Department (data covers the period July 2002-March 2005)

TABLE 3. Job Placement Rates for One-Stop and CFBI Exiters

% of All Served (Count)	WIA Formula Adults	All CFBI Adults	Remedial Care CFBI Adults	Alternative Network CFBI Adults	Specialized Services CFBI Adults
Employed at Exit (All Exiters)	70.4% (17,177)	39.7% (1,347)	22.4% (241)	59.0% (522)	45.2% (230)
	N = 24,389	N = 3,387	N = 1,075	N = 885	N = 509
Employed at Exit (Hardest-to- Employ Exiters)	69.0% (3,058)	37.4% (581)	22.6% (140)	53.7% (204)	41.3% (33)
	N = 4,431	N = 1,553	N = 619	N = 380	N = 80

Source: California Employment Development Department (data covers the period July 2002-March 2005); the hardest-to-employ figures represent the portion of program participants categorized as homeless, ex-offenders, or with substance abuse issues. *Note*: These numbers are based on the 55% of CFBI participants from whom outcomes data is currently available. Since we were not able to definitively classify all CFBI organizations, the numbers reported in remedial care, alternative network, or specialized services categories do not add up to the total for all CFBI adults.

the differences in participant characteristics, we ran a separate comparison of placement rates that was limited to individuals in three hardest-to-employ categories: substance abuse, homeless, and ex-offenders. Even when looking at this subset of the overall population, One-Stop placement rates exceed those of CFBOs, by a margin of 69% to 37%.

A preliminary comparison of CFBO outcomes based on network roles brings into view a more complex pattern of outcomes. This analysis is based on a subset of 23 CFBOs that we are able to code as either remedial care (N = 12), alternative network (N = 8), or specialized service organizations (N = 3).[7] The placement rates for exiters in the remedial care organizations average 22% compared to 45% for those offering specialized services and 59% for the alternative network organizations (Table 3). We suspect that the relatively small 11% gap between alternative network organizations and One-Stops might be even lower than these numbers suggest, given that One-Stops have considerably more experience with managing their clients flows to ensure they meet federal performance standards.

DISCUSSION

A local network perspective presupposes a different kind of methodological rigor that can provide new conceptual insight as researchers assess the effectiveness of faith-based programs and initiatives. Whereas conventional comparative effectiveness evaluations presume that participant outcomes can be linked to stand-alone programs, the network perspective takes seriously the multiplicity of organizations that serve any single individual and the wide range of roles that organizations can play within local service delivery networks. From this vantage point, it becomes clear that participant outcomes are often contingent on the quality of the referral system linking various organizations, and the ability of case managers to help clients navigate among the daunting array of service providers (Alter & Hage, 1993; Mathews & Fawcett, 1981; Wineburg, 2001). As Renz and Herman (2004) have suggested, it may be more appropriate to begin thinking in terms of the concept of "network effectiveness," since the outcomes of value to participants and the public are the products of collaborations that involve many organizations. Wuthnow (2004) also points in this direction, noting that from the participant standpoint what matters is not so much the quality of any particular service they receive, but the overall service portfolio they can assemble from various community resources.

The network perspective can inform an ongoing debate about how faith-based policy initiatives affect the overall performance of local workforce development systems. Some observers express concern that faith-based programs may operate as an "alternative delivery system" that drains money from existing secular nonprofits or government programs in a zero-sum game (Burke, Fossett, & Gais, 2004; Chaves, 2001; Ragan, 2004). Others see the possibility that faith-related organizations may become new partners that advance local goals and complement the efforts of traditional workforce development agencies, particularly if there is careful dialogue about the respective strengths and limits of different organizations (Campbell, 2002; Wineburg, 2001).

Based on our findings, it appears likely that progress in sorting out these issues will depend in part on the ability to carefully distinguish between different types of CFBOs. Remedial care organizations in CFBI excelled in reaching populations that are currently underserved by the workforce development system. Given the right support, most were also able to meet government accountability standards. On the other hand, we found them to be lacking in sophisticated workforce services, and in need of support from more experienced workforce providers to meet participants' needs. The task will be to develop approaches to partnering with these groups that blend their strength in outreach with the job training and placement services present in other community programs.

Alternative network organizations seem especially promising as government partners, and our data confirms that these organizations were more likely to have developed working relationships with One-Stops. While some of these relationships pre-dated CFBI, staff at these CFBOs believe the initiative helped extend and deepen the relationships. Like remedial care organizations, alternative network CFBOs reached many individuals not served by the One-Stop system, and the initial evidence suggests they were nearly as successful as One-Stops in achieving employment outcomes. Further, most alternative network organizations we studied have established track records and deep roots in the community, boding well for their future availability as workforce partners.

Whether special federal or state funding is needed to facilitate CFBO partnerships is an open question. Many remedial care organizations stated that receiving state-level recognition dramatically enhanced their stature in the community, and got them an immediate "seat at the table" in community planning discussions. These same organizations were effusive in praising the role of EDD technical assistance in strengthening their organizational capacity, and also spoke of the benefits of developing connections with their fellow grantees around the state. Finally, we encountered considerable skepticism about faith-based initiatives from many local workforce development officials who might require the spur of a state or federal initiative to give CFBO partnerships a genuine chance.

On the other hand, by organizing these initiatives on a local network basis, rather than primarily via federal or state grants to a single local organization, it might be possible to develop more–and more fruitful–partnerships. Discernments about which organizations could best fill niche roles could be made at the local level, rather than by distant bureaucrats with limited local knowledge and little direct stake in the choices. For example, it may well be possible to establish fruitful connections between One-Stops and remedial care organizations simply by increasing mutual awareness or developing better referral mechanisms, both of which might be accomplished without resorting to a new grant program. Also, the passion and commitment we witnessed among many CFBO directors can be a source of inspirational leadership that can help fuel local collaborations whether or not funding is on the table.

The CFBI case suggests three specific recommendations for state and local policy makers. First, design programs with community development goals in mind, not simply the delivery of individual programs and services. In particular, look for ways to enhance partnerships within local service delivery networks. The use of capacity-building intermediaries as promoted by recent federal initiatives takes a small step in this direction, particularly when government can select intermediaries who themselves work on a community-wide scale and with a broad community development perspective. Or, as in the CFBI case, government agencies can seek to reinvent themselves in a manner that treats community intervention as a holistic process rather than as a series of discrete grants and programs with little attention to inter-organizational relationships.

Second, carefully distinguish between the type of remedial services and relational care that are the primary offering of many CFBOs, and the funding of more substantive educational and job training services. It will not help local communities if a "thousand points of light" blossom only to see educational opportunities in the first-chance and second-chance systems systematically under-funded and allowed to languish. Communities need ways to mobilize moral support and encouragement, but not if it comes at the expense of distracting attention from the critical need for other forms of public investment.

Finally, ensure that research into faith-based initiatives combines both process and outcomes evaluation, moving beyond the conventions underlying many efforts to assess comparative effectiveness. Evaluative studies often carry the conceptual baggage of a competitive market model, in which the issue is how to ensure that government funding goes to the most efficient and effective providers. When the network becomes the unit of analysis, and network effectiveness is the key variable, policy choices can take shape based on a more realistic understanding of how services are actually delivered within communities, and how those services are experienced by program participants. What is needed is not information on which to base competitive contracting decisions, but the type of local knowledge that facilitates longer-term partnership development and makes use of the full range of community assets. Researchers can help inform this community change process, but will need to move beyond traditional approaches to evaluation in order to become more useful (Auspos & Kubisch, 2004).

NOTES

1. In May 2002, California's Employment Development Department's Audit and Evaluation Division (A&ED) organized a research consortium that included researchers at two California State University campuses (Humboldt and San Bernardino), the University of California, Davis, and three state entities (the Employment Development Department, the Health and Human Services Agency, and the Labor and Workforce Development Agency). A total of $250,000 was allocated for the work of the research

consortium. An additional $250,000 allocation was made by EDD to the UC Davis team to conduct a second phase of the evaluation, featuring a community network analysis. The views in this article reflect the work and conclusions of the UC Davis research team, and the contributions of EDD in providing administrative data analysis, and do not necessarily reflect the views of the other members of the research consortium. However, we would like to acknowledge the contributions of Shel Bockman, Judith Little, and Barbara W. Sirotnik to the overall project.

2. Using state general funds, 20 organizations received their initial funding during the 2000-01 fiscal year. The following year another 20 organizations were selected and funding for all 40 organizations shifted to federal Workforce Investment Act (WIA) dollars available through the Governor's 15% discretionary funds. The initial round of funding was made available only to faith-related nonprofits. After a lawsuit was filed challenging this practice, the second competitive grant process was opened to any 501(c)3 organization.

3. Until budget cuts at EDD curtailed travel, the capacity building effort included twice monthly visits by program managers to CFBI organizations. Program managers not only worked to ensure that funded organizations met formal reporting requirements, they also assisted newer organizations with basic nonprofit development concerns, sometimes by identifying appropriate organizational consultants. Funded organizations were highly satisfied with the EDD effort, which they did not expect from a government program.

4. Based on coding of the scoping surveys, we used six years longevity as the dividing line between newer and more established organizations.

5. We were unable to complete interviews with two of the 30 faith-based organizations.

6. As a demonstration program, CFBI-funded organizations were considered exempt from federal performance standards during the project.

7. Pending an analysis of an ongoing back-end survey of the CFBI-funded organizations, we eventually expect to be able to code more of the 40 CFBOs and conduct a more definitive analysis.

REFERENCES

Alter, C., & Hage, J. (1993). *Organizations Working Together.* Newbury Park: Sage Publications.

Auspos, P., & Kubisch, A.C. (2004). Building Knowledge about Community Change: Moving Beyond Evaluations. The Aspen Institute, Roundtable on Community Change.

Brustein, M., & Knight, R. (1998). A Guide to the Workforce Investment Act. The National Association of Private Industry Councils.

Burke, C., Fossett, J., & Gais, T. (October 2004). Funding Faith-Based Services in a Time of Fiscal Pressures. Albany, NY: Rockefeller Institute of Government.

Campbell, D. (2002). Beyond Charitable Choice: The Diverse Service Delivery Approaches of Local Faith-Related Organizations. *Nonprofit and Voluntary Sector Quarterly*, 31(2), 207-230.

Chaves, M. (2001). Going on Faith. *Christian Century*, 118(25), 20.

Cisneros, H.G. (1996). *Higher Ground: Faith Communities and Community Building.* Washington, DC: U.S. Department of Housing and Urban Development.

Cnaan, R.A., with Wineburg, R.J., & Boddie, S.C. (2000). *The Newer Deal: Social Work and Religion in Partnership.* New York: Columbia University Press.

Deb, P., & Jones, D. (October 2003). Does Faith Work? A Comparison of Labor Market Outcomes of Religious and Secular Job Training Programs. Center for Urban Policy and the Environment, School of Public and Environmental Affairs, Indiana University–Purdue University Indianapolis.

Franklin, G., & Ripley, R.B. (1984). *CETA: Politics and Policy 1973-1982.* Knoxville: University of Tennessee Press.

Glenn, C.L. (2000). *The Ambiguous Embrace: Government and Faith-Based Schools and Social Agencies.* Princeton: Princeton University Press.

Green, J.C., & Sherman, A.L. (2002). Fruitful Collaborations: A Survey of Government-Funded Faith-Based Programs in 15 State. Fishers, Indiana: The Hudson Institute.

Gutek, B.A. (1995). *The Dynamics of Service.* San Francisco: Jossey-Bass Publishers.

Harrison, B., & Weiss, M. (1998). *Workforce Development Networks: Community-Based Organizations and Regional Alliances.* Thousand Oaks, CA: Sage Publications.

Johnson, B.R. (2002). Objective Hope Assessing the Effectiveness of Faith-Based Organizations: A Review of the Literature. Center for Research on Religion and Urban Civil Society.

Kramer, F.D., & Nightingale D.S. et al. (2002). Faith-Based Organizations Providing Employment and Training Services: A Preliminary Exploration. The Urban Institute.

Magnum, G.L. (2000). Reflections on Training Policies and Programs, in *Improving the Odds: Increasing the Effectiveness of Publicly Funded Training* (pp. 293-332). Washington, DC: The Urban Institute.

Mathews, M.R., & Fawcett, S.B. (1981). Matching Clients and Services: Information and Referral. Beverly Hills: Sage Publications.

Monsma, S.V. with Mounts, C.M. (2002). Working Faith: How Religious Organizations Provide Welfare-to-Work Services. Center for Research on Religion and Urban Civil Society.

Moore, M.H. (1995). Creating Public Value: Strategic Management in Government. Cambridge, MA: Harvard University Press.

Ragan, M. (October 2004). Faith-based vs. Secular: Using Administrative Data to Compare the Performance of Faith-Affiliated and Other Social Service Providers. Albany, NY: Rockefeller Institute of Government.

Renz, D.O., & Herman, R.D. (2004). More Theses on Nonprofit Effectiveness. *ARNOVA News*, 33(4), 10-11.

Sherman, A.L. (2002). Reinvigorating Faith in Communities. Fishers, IN: The Hudson Institute.

Smith, S.R., & Sosin, M.R. (2001). The Varieties of Faith-Related Agencies. *Public Administration Review*, 61(6), 651-670.

Wineburg, R. (2001). *A Limited Partnership: The Politics of Religion, Welfare, and Social Service*. NY: Columbia University Press.

Wuthnow, R. 2004. *Saving America? Faith-Based Services and the Future of Civil Society*. Princeton, NJ: Princeton University Press.

Chapter 13

Belief Systems
in Faith-Based Human Service Programs

F. Ellen Netting
Mary Katherine O'Connor
Gaynor Yancey

F. Ellen Netting, PhD, is Professor, Virginia Commonwealth University School
of Social Work, 1001 West Franklin Street, Richmond, VA 23284-2027 (E-mail:
enetting@vcu.edu). Mary Katherine O'Connor, PhD, is Professor, Virginia Commonwealth University School of Social Work, 1001 West Franklin Street, Richmond, VA
23284-2027 (E-mail: mkoconno@vcu.edu). Gaynor Yancey, DSW, is Assistant Professor, Baylor University School of Social Work, One Bear Place #97320, Waco, TX
76798-7320 (E-mail: Gaynor_Yancey@ baylor.edu).
This project is funded by a generous grant from The Pew Charitable Trusts. Special
appreciation to members of the Faith & Service Technical Education Network
(FASTEN) Team at Baylor University, University of Pittsburgh, University of Southern California, and Virginia Commonwealth University who collected the data in
Phase I on which this article is based.
The findings of this first phase is the foundation for a quantitative national survey
designed to determine the extent to which the grounded theory that emerges in the project's first phase can be applied nationally across the diversity of faith-based social services in the United States. The Hudson Institute and the Center for Faith and Service of
the National Crime Prevention Council (NCPC), Baylor's partners in this project, are
disseminating the findings of this research through FASTEN.

[Haworth co-indexing entry note]: "Belief Systems in Faith-Based Human Service Programs." Netting,
F. Ellen, Mary Katherine O'Connor, and Gaynor Yancey. Co-published simultaneously in *Journal of Reli-
gion & Spirituality in Social Work* (The Haworth Pastoral Press, an imprint of The Haworth Press, Inc.) Vol. 25,
No. 3/4, 2006, pp. 261-286; and: *Faith-Based Social Services: Measures, Assessments, and Effectiveness* (ed:
Stephanie C. Boddie, and Ram A. Cnaan) The Haworth Pastoral Press, an imprint of The Haworth Press, Inc.,
2006, pp. 261-286.

SUMMARY. Using a grounded theory design and methods, 65 key informants in 15 faith-based organizations having promising programs in four urban areas were interviewed. Respondents were asked what makes their direct service programs faith-based. A story emerges, motivated by mission-driven visions tied to forces beyond local programs and steeped in deep traditions. A major implication of the findings is that in teaching people about the various practices of diverse religious groups, we are only giving them the visible elements. While the expressed values of acts and faith are integral in the faith-based discussion, they do not tell the full story. The deep drivers of human behavior and practice are found in the specific beliefs and interpretations of individuals who are involved either as leaders or participants in faith-based organizations. For many of these individuals in faith-based organizations, mission and accountability to God trumps secular or professional expectations. doi:10.1300/J377v25n03_15

KEYWORDS. Grounded theory, faith-based organizations, social services, religion, organizational culture

An accelerated public focus on *faith-based* services has highlighted an entangled political, religious, ideological, cultural, economic, and social context in which human services are provided (Cnaan, 1999; Stoesen, 2004; Wineburg, 2001). Attempts to clarify, define, and understand faith-based initiatives have spurred the creation of The Roundtable on Religion and Social Welfare Policy, various typologies (Goggins & Orth, 2002; Jeavons, 1997; Monsma, 1996; Sider & Unruh, 2004), professional meetings and conferences, funding opportunities, and increasing interdisciplinary research on every conceivable aspect of the subject. In an attempt to connect what is known about management in human service organizations to persons working in faith-based organizations, a growing number of books have been written over the last decade (Brinckerhoff, 1999; Holland & Hester, 2000; Jeavons & Basinger, 1995; Queen, 2000). The faith-based dialogue is long established, albeit much more in the public eye in recent years. It promises to continue as an important leg of the journey in comprehending the character of the voluntary or nonprofit sector in the United States.

Human service programs are delivered under various auspices. Those that are "faith-based" can be attached to congregations, grassroots associations, and/or nonprofit organizations. Their structural arrangements appear to be as varied as one can imagine within the parameters of state corporation law. It is not just faith-based programs about which questions are raised. The entire nonprofit sector, in its broadest definition, is viewed as engaged in an ongoing crisis of identity (Salamon, 2002). Advice on how to resolve this identity crisis is debated (Lewis, 2002; Minkoff, 2002) as tensions between providing services and promoting broader scale community or even societal change are examined in the nonprofit literature (Campbell, 2002; Hyde, 2000; Koroloff & Briggs, 1996). Therefore, dialogue about faith-based organizations and their programs are set within a nonprofit context in which the very nature of the voluntary sector is under scrutiny.

In this paper, we begin with selected insights from the literature in an attempt to put our paper in context. We follow with an overview of the study, then report results that have emerged in the process of extensive interviews with persons involved in diverse service delivery roles in geographically-dispersed, exemplary faith-based programs in the United States. The research question is "what makes your program faith-based?" Results reveal how the motivational depth of belief systems across faith traditions appears to influence every aspect of service delivery at the program level. We end with implications for social science in general and for practitioner understanding in particular.

THE VALUE-EXPRESSIVE ASPECT
OF HUMAN SERVICE ORGANIZATIONS

A huge literature on organizational culture has emerged over the last two decades, recognizing the value-expressive nature of organizations (Frost, Moore, Louis, Lundberg, & Martin, 1991; Martin, 2002; Ott, 1989; Schein, 1992; Shultz, 1995). In the management, business, and sociological literature, there have been studies of hundreds of businesses that reveal the paradoxes posed by competing values within organizational life (Cameron & Quinn, 1999; Quinn, 1989). It is not surprising then that in human service organizations, in which human beings are the products, the nature of the work is value-expressive. Hasenfeld (2000) frames it well when he says, "human service organizations engage in moral work, upholding and reinforcing moral values about 'desirable' human behavior and the 'good society'" (p. 90).

Jeavons (1992) has been particularly articulate in examining the value-expressive character of nonprofit agencies. He focuses on their historical roots as social welfare services were considered "the business of the church because they could be undertaken as an expression of religious calling and religious tenets" (p. 404). He argues that "it is precisely the values-expressive nature of religious, philanthropic work and the agencies engaged in it, that created social space in which an independent sector could form . . ." (p. 404). Scholars such as Jeavons (1992) and Chambre (2001) indicate that the value-expressive nature of nonprofit organizations must be acknowledged if one is to comprehend fully the complexity and understand the difference between nongovernmental organizations (NGOs) and business models. The value-expressive nature of nonprofit organizations is particularly relevant for those that consider themselves "faith-based."

Other writers have focused on the importance of the roots (Billis, 1991) and traditions (Queen, 2000) of nonprofit organizations. For example, Milofsky (1997) sees tradition as "especially noteworthy as symbols or icons that call forth images both of what the work is and how in its most virtuous form it is carried out" (p. 261). Milofsky points out that commitment is inspired through tradition and that a tradition requires a collective of others with whom passion can be shared. Thus, an inexplicable pattern of behavior may, indeed, be a "tradition."

Queen (2000) contends "that religious traditions combine a commitment to community with a commitment to the inherent worth of individuals [thus providing] a focal point for the increasing attention paid to the role of religiously based human and social services" (p. 12). Sider and Unruh (2004), in their recently developed typology, acknowledge the value-expressive nature, the roots, and traditions of faith-based organizations. They focus explicitly on "visibly expressive ways" in which religion may be present for two reasons. First, these factors are easier to observe and verify than deep underlying subjective meanings. They explain that to delve further would require in-depth interviews with various representatives in order to fully explore underlying religious beliefs and motivations. Second, their focus is on public policy and the debate on faith-based initiatives. The more visible elements of religious expression are the most controversial because they are most obvious (e.g., hiring practices, religious services, etc.).

Rogers, Yancey, Singletary, Garland, and Brennan Homiak (2006) have found through their F.A.S.T.E.N. research study that there is a difference in faith identity and faith culture and that this difference may impact the provision of services in faith-based programs. *Faith identity* refers not only to an organization's historic religious purposes and connections, but also to its current motivation and mission. An organization's faith identity then could include its program's faith goals for participants such as: spiritual development, religious conversion, positive change through prayer, moral living, social and economic justice, or an introduction to worship. *Faith culture,* on the other hand, is related to the expression of faith in an organization or congregation. The "Faith Scale" they have created from the emerging data from respondents identifies how the organization incorporates faith on a daily basis in its hiring practices, measures for success, and service delivery. For some organizations, faith is an explicit criterion for hiring staff and management, but for others it is only implicit or does not play an explicit role. Similarly, some organizations use faith as a criterion for measuring success; for example, organizations in the study ranked how important spiritual transformation/improvement of participants was in determining success of services. The faith content in services is another important measure of faith culture that reveals whether faith activities are mandatory, invitational, or not even present. An organization that has a strong faith culture usually has a more explicit and well-defined expression of faith in terms of hiring, faith content for participants, and success criteria for the program.

In the study that follows, social service programs were intentionally selected. Respondents were asked what makes their direct service programs faith-based. The organizations within which these programs are housed are influenced by guiding philosophies, belief systems, traditions and values. A story emerges, motivated by mission-driven visions tied to forces beyond local programs and steeped in deep traditions.

THE STUDY

In Spring 2002, the Pew Charitable Trusts awarded a grant to the Baylor University School of Social Work to conduct research designed to identify factors that contribute to the effectiveness of faith-based programs in addressing problems of urban poverty. Baylor's School of Social Work was joined by researchers from Baylor's business school, the schools of social work at the University of Pittsburgh and Virginia Commonwealth University, and the Center for Religion and Civic Culture at the University of Southern California.

The full project is a grounded theory approach comprised of three phases. The first phase was qualitative and emergent following a Strauss and Corbin (1998) model. The results of the first phase (a part of which is reported here) became the structure for a questionnaire on promising faith-based programs on a national sample that was part of phase 2. As a triangulation for the quantitative data, a second round of qualitative interviews were also undertaken in the same metropolitan areas where the questionnaires were distributed following the same structure as the quantitative instrument. The final phase involves production of reports of all phases of this multi-method project.

A team of researchers from the four universities interviewed various stakeholders from promising faith-based programs in four United States regions for Phase 1 of the grounded theory design. This involved in-depth qualitative interviews with 65 key informants in selected programs (Strauss & Corbin, 1998). A purposive sample of 15 organizations having "promising programs" in four urban areas was selected. Promising programs were those identified by local community members as being innovative and successful. Every attempt was made to obtain maximum variation among all sites in the selection process along the dimensions of structure, funding source(s), and service population(s), and with special attention to racial diversity, intensity of collaboration, degree of professionalism/formality, stage of organizational development, and religious/faith orientation. Direct service intervention programs were deliberately selected rather than the numerous advocacy and community development programs sponsored by faith-based groups because it is through direct service interventions that the immediate needs of people are addressed. It also created an opportunity to interview participants (clients) who could tell us about their experiences with the program. Semi-structured interview guides were used to ask an average of five stakeholders in each program, representing the following roles: program administrators, staff members, participants/clients, board members, and collaborators what makes programs faith-based. Respondents were encouraged to tell us whatever they wanted to tell us about this aspect of their programs. ATLAS.ti, a qualitative software package, was used to analyze the recorded and transcribed interviews using the constant comparison method (Glaser & Strauss, 1967; O'Connor, 2002; Weiss, 1994) and producing networks representing all the concepts and themes that emerged.

Of the 15 programs studied in Phase 1, 11 were housed in religiously affiliated 501(c) (3) organizations and 4 were located in congregations. All were located in large urban areas and all served persons with low incomes. Nine (9) were related to Protestant denominations, whereas 2 were Catholic, 2 were Muslim, 1 was Jewish, and 1 was Interfaith. Programs ranged in age with 3 being new (1 year), 6 being middle-aged (up to 4 years old), and 6 being mature (5 years or older). Programs served diverse groups, including African-American, Anglo, Native American, Latino, Bi-Racial, Jewish, Somali, Afghani, Moroccan, Kosovar, and Kurdish people. Services provided through these diverse programs included education, counseling, treatment, housing, resettlement, foster care, health care, and job development.

Many themes emerged in the process of these numerous interviews. Therefore, the focus of the findings reported below is on the impact of the belief systems within these promising programs and what makes them faith-based. Other findings from other networks from Phase 1 are discussed elsewhere (Netting, O'Connor, Thomas, & Yancey, 2005; Yancey & Atkinson, 2004).

FINDINGS

It is important to emphasize that the findings reported here cannot be generalized to other programs. The purpose of grounded theory research is to ground findings in context by listening to the voices of respondents (in this study, that included hearing from selected program participants, the clients, as well as organizational members) and to allow the theory to unfold from their experiences in such a way as to allow for further testing in other contexts. Thus, as different and unique as each program studied is, a type of similarity emerges as respondents talk about what makes their programs faith-based. Whether programs are large or small, young or old, being faith-based appears to tie respondents to guiding philosophies deeply embedded in traditions far beyond the scope of the programs themselves. A story emerges that transcends geographic site and, sometimes, even religious tradition. As a staff member in a Texas program put it, "our motivation . . . permeates the whole philosophy of the program . . . [clients] take with them something that can never be taken from them . . . it won't be lost anywhere."

We begin by focusing on the less visible ways in which sets of beliefs guide faith-based organizations and their programs, the philosophies and traditions that are part of the select group of organizations under study. Persons who are part of the religious traditions represented here (Christian, Jewish, and Muslim) are motivated by moral imperatives to serve and beliefs that they are accountable to God. This finding is not surprising because the call to service emanates from mono-theistic faith traditions whose roots are intricately tied. Thus, respondent voices are remarkably similar in describing their calls to perform acts of service and to please God, even though the nuances of evangelical language will differ. There are broad commonalities that obscure the differences in how these overriding beliefs are carried out in practice. Thus, the great traditions of the groups studied are somewhat compatible in their guiding philosophies.

These great traditions are reflected in the study themes called (1) Moral Imperatives to Serve, and (2) Accountability to God. Tied to Accountability to God are themes and lessons learned about the Influence of Mission on Operations, and the importance of Founders, Tradition, and Religious Writings as ways of deeply embedding these traditions in the organization and programmatic culture (see Figure 1). It is noteworthy that the typology suggested here is similar to Max Weber's classical dual authority concept; however, the nuanced richness of these findings provides a typological depth new to the social science literature.

Moral Imperatives to Serve

A Texas Baptist staff member refers to the spiritual component of their program as a "moral imperative." Muslims, Jews, and Christians

FIGURE 1. Belief System Influence on Faith-Based Human Service Programs

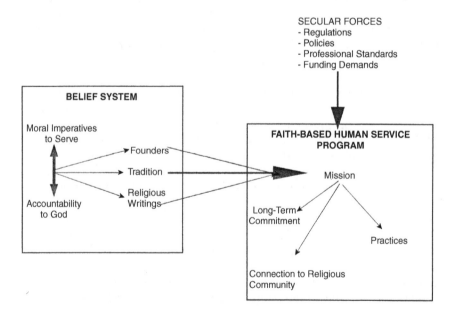

talk about their traditions as guiding them to serve others. Whereas a Christian staff member calls it making a "difference in the future . . . and having the opportunity to impact generations we'll never see," a California-based Muslim collaborator says that in order to serve God, "when Muslims give back to the community [they must] give and give and give." Similarly, a Jewish staff member in Pennsylvania talks about the motivation felt in serving others. "It's been just an incredible experience for me as a Jew working with these folks because this is to me what it is to be a faith-based organization, to be able to provide services to people who have had such horrendous experiences . . . were totally tormented, tortured and their families killed just because they were Jewish." Describing a congregationally-based Christian program, an administrator in California ponders the concept of service, saying that if "we can't service [clients], we can't leave them empty-handed because, before we are a social service agency, we are [a church]. And because we're [the church] we have to honor the oath of the spiritual realm, which is service."

Thus, the call to perform service cannot be ignored even if the appropriate service is not available to the person in need. Empty-handedness is not an option because some response is demanded by the faith-based nature of the program. A Texas-based program administrator continues, "We will help you find wherever it is you need to belong. And if it's not here . . . we will hook you up to wherever you need to be." A staff member in the same program explains that "we try to find out what is your passion, what did God create you to do." Another administrator in a different Texas program comments that "mission is more important than the operation of the organization itself and our values are supported by our faith in working with the individuals toward a goal of assisting them towards self-sufficiency." In a California-based program, an administrator explains, "So for me, I keep that model in my head; if I help someone, then not only have I done a great deed, but I've pleased God . . . I was raised to believe that if I can help someone along the way, then my living shall not be in vain."

Accountability to God

This accountability to God, to a higher calling, to a being beyond oneself is evident across traditions. The call to serve transcends the program or organization in which the service is provided. It is described as externally derived, usually from God. A Christian staff member talks about serving the total person. "When you understand the Word of God, you learn how to do it." A Muslim administrator says that the creation of the program is an "attempt to really embody the true understandings of why this religion was revealed to mankind . . . we don't ask [for a] reward from anybody except God. That's what it comes down to, and that is the basic tenet of our faith." Staff members in multiple locations use phrases throughout the interview data like "I'm a Christian, so I prayed. . . . What do you want me to do, Lord?" or "it's what God has planned for me" or "God has a plan" or "this is God's program . . . we really don't do anything without consulting God first. God can even have Plans 'A' & 'B.' " A staff member in a California-based child welfare program states, "We have families that go into this knowing that God didn't put that child with them in the first place. That it's not their child. And God's Plan A is for the child to go back if that family heals."

Influence of Mission on Operations

The accountability to a higher being influences what people do in these programs. If the line to a higher being such as God is paramount, then responsibilities to professional standards, policies, and even administrative or ecclesiastical directives may be less important than pleasing God. For example, a Pennsylvania-based staff member talks about how professionals may actually constrain client potential for growth and development by working closely with existing secular systems in reviewing cases and dealing with court officials.

Respondents are aware of the balance they must achieve in being accountable to God as well as to secular sources. One Texas staff member explains it this way: "I believe that all of us work out of a spirituality of our own, that there is a sense of a Higher Being in our life. We're not the end all and be all of what is, there is something bigger. And so we believe that there is God, in whatever form that may be. And that influences the way we perceive our folks, that we see the godliness in those around us . . . I think our investments are different [from government], our ways of dealing with people are different." A collaborator with a Muslim based nonprofit in California says that it "is not really different because it's a Muslim organization . . . certainly there are certain things about Muslim philosophy that might come into play . . ." A Virginia-based administrator recognizes that "a lot of time and effort is spent on hard things, perhaps boring things, but things that have to happen for innovation and creativity." However, an administrator in Texas acknowledges that "the mission is more important than the operation of the organization itself and that our values are supported by our faith in working with the individuals toward a goal of assisting them towards self-sufficiency." Leaving things "in His hands" indicates God is the ultimate director. According to a staff member in Pennsylvania "maybe [He's] the extra push in the intangible willingness to adopt and make things work, it's not written in stone, but it's just there . . . Yeah, we need [the funding source] to be happy because [they] are going to write the check, but our calling is higher." A California-based staff person says "I don't think that it's that the secular community can't. I just don't think that they do. I don't think that their heart is there . . . we feel called by God to do this."

Founders

This higher calling motivated the founders of the organizations. Wosh (2004) addresses the importance of founders in his work, *Covenant House: Journey of a Faith-Based Charity*. Like his work, we found that legends evolve around how they set up the organizations in which these programs are housed, maintaining a commitment to a God-driven mission. A Catholic staff person in Pennsylvania speaks of the nuns who founded their organization and the strength of their influence, no matter how many of the Sisters are physically present today. Recounting how a nun oriented them to their history, she says "you could see where our organization and the Sisters, being faith-based, why we do the things we do for the poor and for the vulnerable, like never giving up or working really hard on never giving up. And I think that's rooted in [our history] and in our future." A Protestant female physician founded a shelter program when "she saw babies in cribs in the hallways and it broke her heart. She said 'where are the churches? . . . [and] she went to them." The story continues that she and her spouse (an attorney) set up the program in their garage to begin its operation.

Tradition

Organizations in which programs are housed are seen as having deep roots in accountability to their faith traditions. Participants from a California-based Muslim organization, seen as the first of its kind, relate how persons of the Muslim faith look for guidance from the organization. One administrator says, "It was to show mercy in the making. And so, what makes it unique is that a lot of Muslims will agree . . . [it] becomes an icon for Muslim social service instantly because it's just never been done before." In a similar response, a Christian respondent replies "we are rooted in history and tradition here. We are very much a faith-based organization; we don't deny it; we don't hide it; and we put it out there in the forefront. This is a Catholic organization." A Jewish respondent reveals "The first thing I think people set up were burial societies to bury their dead. And then other things, social services grew from that. And so it was very much faith-based. It was very much centered in the Jewish community. It was helping immigrants resettling here, providing counseling, you know the whole nine yards." Revealing the depth of tradition based in accountability to God, an administrator shares a personal reflection, "If you don't have your roots, you don't have anything. You need to be helping someone . . . this is not only my job, but this is my destiny."

Religious Writings

Entire rationales for programs are built on religious text. For example, a board member of a Virginia-based program targeting African American men indicates that the program is based on "the last book in the Old Testament. The last verse talks about God going to turn the heart of the fathers back toward their children and the heart of their children back toward their fathers . . . when a man is out of place, you have the whole nation out of place. So until the man gets back into his home, and to raise his kids, our nation will never be right." The administrator describes the program as "hope restored."

Combining what is said about accountability to God, whether it is through mission, tradition, founders or religious writings, respondents agree that they are directed from a source beyond themselves. One respondent summed it up by saying "we know who we are."

Faith-Based Practices

Similar abstract language, based in similar guiding philosophies, generates a diversity of interpretations about what appropriately constitutes faith-based service. From the theological/philosophical overview just presented, it becomes clear that though the descriptions of the respondents' calls to serve and accountability to God are similar, there is great divergence in how this call is carried out. As closely tied as respondents are when they describe their calls and perceptions of accountability, their divergence is increasingly obvious as they talk about what makes their direct practice faith-based (Rogers et al., 2006). The following themes emerge: Long-Term Commitment, Connection with Faith Community, and Practices.

Long-Term Commitment

If staff perceive that a higher being calls them to perform the mission of service, then the commitment to perform in a consistent and long-term manner seems equally imperative. A staff person working for a Baptist program used words such as we "make a difference in the future" or have the opportunity "to impact a generation that we'll never see . . . the most important and special part is that we have the opportunity to introduce [service recipients] to the Creator of the universe . . . to impact a life for eternity." This long-term impact is reflected in programs in different locations. An administrator in a Catholic program talks about "long lasting results" and what it takes to "sustain change." Other respondents refer to "trying to break the cycle of homelessness," seeing the "big picture," looking out for the "next generation." An administrator in a United Methodist program for children remarks, "Everyone is told from the day they come in the organization that we attempt "to touch a life and create a future."

Relationally, long-term commitment requires stamina in sticking with clients when others might give up. Talking about the commitment of foster families recruited through local congregations, one respondent says, "I know if their hearts weren't dedicated to what God wanted them to do, [they] would have called the social worker and said, we are so done with this. True commitment is that we are called. It doesn't matter what the child does, what the child steals or what the biological parents are putting us through or what the system is putting us through. We, through prayer and through our friends' support, are committing to this child. And it's like being married and divorced, saying divorce is not an option." Calling and long-term commitment seem to go hand-in-hand. "So we're not really fly-by-night people with a wild idea, you know, I'm just going to give this a shot and if it doesn't work . . . we don't consider these children just cargo or, you know just baggage . . . they are lives!" From another program in a different part of the country, a voice echoes the belief that, "there's no one who is hopeless, that there is no one who should be the marginalized of our society."

Connection with Faith Community

The value in being connected to a religious community that has an existing structure and a cadre of committed people is emphasized throughout the interviews. These are not isolated programs in local communities; they are networked within their religious traditions. These ties appear to strengthen the level of commitment. Four programs are actually based in congregations that have an established association of members who participate in the life of the program.

Most service-providing respondents indicate that they are open to serving people of all religious backgrounds and beliefs, but some faith-based organizations or organizational leaders that have traditions steeped in evangelism (converting souls) suggest some struggle with this openness, particularly with persons who are not part of any religious tradition. In a California-based program that is open to diverse religious traditions, a client explains how social workers from their program who come from the same denomination are sent into local churches to recruit volunteers and request funds because they are seen as being "from a church." Anyone else would still be seen as "an outsider." Meanwhile, in a Virginia-based program, a staff member smiles as she talks about persons applying for staff positions who have the same religious affiliation as the organization; "it's almost like extra credit. It gives them points, but it's not a question we ever ask."

A Jewish staff member in Pennsylvania tells a story. "When I go into someone's home who's Jewish . . . they'll say a Yiddish word and 'Do you know what that means?' and I'll say 'yeah." And they'll say 'oh are you Jewish?' And I'll say 'Yeah.' and immediately, it's almost like this connection is made like I understand who they are, where they come from, what they've been through, and they understand that I understand that." A Texas staff person talks about how clients are often invited "into their churches to go and worship with them." A California administrator adds, "I think what the faith community adds to the mix is a commitment to personal relationships because that really is a sense of community which is at the heart of every faith community."

The connection to a faith community is often expressed through language and symbols. Visibly expressive language, symbols, and activities are present in most programs and within the organizations that sponsor them. Freedom to engage in "God-talk" or religious sounding language is part of program culture that is practiced without apology. In fact, respondents reveal how important it is to be in a place in which the norms allow one to talk about God or their own spirituality. Being tied to a faith community of some sort is described by a Texas-based program administrator as having "a relational element," as allowing one to build relationships, and to connect with others.

Building relationships with the faith community can be overt. Referring to children who participate in a very long-established program in a 100 years old Virginia-based faith-based organization, a client explains,

"You are really teaching them morals . . . that's what I can say about faith . . . knowing that we are here to support you, and showing you the right way to go, and talking about what is right and what is wrong and that sort of thing." Socialization to the faith community's value system is explicit in the teaching of morals. A staff person in a different Virginia organization talks about how faith values are transmitted by the artifacts with which she surrounds herself. Pointing around the office, she says, "I've got St. Louise here and an angel there, the patron saint of social workers, and then I've got this mother and child photo and a little angel there. You know it's not something that I talk about, but they're here." Another respondent, a client in a Texas-based Protestant agency, talks about why the agency tried not to have too many artifacts in plain view. "They want this place to be home to everybody and that spirituality is a human condition, not a religious condition. In my view, they recognize that appropriately and provide services to anyone who seeks [them]." Additionally, a Jewish staff member in Pennsylvania talks about cultural artifacts being as relevant as those that are considered religious.

Practices

As respondents talk about connections with religious communities, as well as the language and artifacts of their respective faith traditions, conversations focus on those visually expressive activities that reflect their larger faith traditions. The daily manifestation of being called to serve, of being accountable to God, and of maintaining long-term commitments begins to move toward more specific phenomenon, all within the dialogue about what makes their programs faith-based. As this dialogue moves, so does the divergence among interviewees, each offering their own perspectives about what is appropriate and inappropriate as expressions of faith in practice and action.

Protestant respondents form a continuum of perspectives about the appropriateness of sharing one's faith through visual expressions. At least two such programs refuse to accept government funds because they limit the ability to evangelize. Christian programs are particularly conversant about putting faith into action through prayer, and evangelical Christian programs are unapologetic about it. A Protestant staff member in California says, "But we are going to open our meetings with prayer and you're not . . . you can definitely be a member if you're a Jew or a Morman or a nothing, you know. But you do need to know who we are." In a program that focuses on women's needs, another respondent explains how "we are free to share our faith; we are able to try to get these ladies to accept Christ. I mean we are free to do that and we don't want anything to happen to that freedom."

Protestant programs reveal methods in which prayer becomes a vehicle for witnessing, for putting their faith into action. The concept of a prayer walk is described by one respondent as going to the location in which program participants are attending classes and then walking through the various rooms and observing activities, praying as they are walking. As one Protestant staff member indicates "whether that is verbally or silently just praying through the day [about] what a woman would go through in that building. Just praying on her behalf and praying on behalf of the ministry itself." Prayer is offered in various staff meetings in different programs. "The staff in our program practices their faith. We will oftentimes start our meetings, staff meetings, with a prayer. So the residents in our program sometimes observe us practicing our faith. But we in no way impose on them as mandatory their participation in any type of religious activity." This same respondent adds that program staff members "do look at every piece of literature that we display. And there have been rare instances where we might not want to display a piece of literature only because we felt that it might be offensive to someone in some way or might be disrespectful to them . . . so that is somewhat subjective." Additionally, as respondents in more evangelical Christian traditions are interviewed, they reveal ways in which local churches work with them to provide Bible studies. A Texas program client explains how such classes "teach them how to think differently and approach problems differently than what they've been taught or are used to." Called to witness their faith, the administrator in that same program reveals how "In the book of James it says I will show you my faith by what I do. That is what we do."

Conversely, though, a less evangelical Protestant staff person in Texas talks about discouraging "local churches that come in to entertain from witnessing because that's a captive audience." A staff person in a Virginia program explains that "you can't just totally dump your faith on [clients] . . . one of the things I realized when God [through] Jesus, wanted to save the world, he stepped down from heaven; he came down to the world that we were living in and walked among us and began to, so that we could touch and feel it, and he felt our pain . . ." This program that focuses on the needs of African American men realizes that dumping faith may actually alienate rather than help.

Joining Protestant respondents who are less prone to overt evangelism are Catholic respondents. In one child-serving program, a staff member explains "you can talk about it without kinda pushing one belief system on them, but helping them to see that as a resource." A client in the same Catholic program makes a distinction between evangelism with a big "E" and evangelism with a little "e." "Big 'E' evangelism tends to be in your face . . . explicit witnessing. The sort of evangelization that goes on with [this program] is more small 'e' evangelization–a focus on values, a focus on social justice, a focus on fundamental fairness, civility, providing a safe place for kids." Hundreds of miles away, an administrator in a different Pennsylvania-based Catholic program muses, "We are faith-based, but it's not that we're in the business of proselytizing or converting, but at the same time, we don't hide our Catholic foundation . . . yet we respect all beliefs and religions . . . when you show up here it's out there in the forefront, you see it and we are not trying to hide it." This same respondent adds the importance of recognizing staff religious needs, adding "I don't know of very many social service organizations that allow staff members to take a half hour out of their work schedule and go to chapel and do either quiet reflection or talk about beliefs and frustrations and their relationship with Jesus Christ."

Jewish and Muslim respondents are less evangelically oriented in their responses. A Jewish staff person in Pennsylvania explains, "When you start talking faith-based, it's like what are you talking about? Our organization is really non-sectarian. I mean, we'll work with anyone. And we're not going to preach to them anything in particular. But I think when you go to other faith-based organizations, they will." A Muslim respondent in California indicates that the way in which witnessing occurs is that "we don't have to say anything [like] 'please ask us about Islam' because people see it through our actions."

Throughout the interviews, explicit faith-based practices are discussed. Religious education services, chaplaincy services, community ministry coordination positions, use of staff from local congregations, spiritual enrichment components, the name and history of the organization in which the program is located, the founder's vision grounded in faith, the membership of the board, the ownership of property, even the current administrator's ties to a faith tradition–all become artifacts in the program's culture. The variation is distinctive depending on how evangelical the program leaders are, yet every program has some grounding in the elements of their religious tradition. Inherent in the comments are references to the unique quality of being faith-based. An administrator in a Pennsylvania Catholic agency says, "[Clients] can go to a non-faith-based human service agency, but the folks that have applied here, and they will tell you, there's something unique about the mission and the values and the way that folks interact and are treated here. I think that's what makes us unique and very special." To be definitive about what is unique about the mission, the values, and the practices of these faith-based organizations is challenging, at best. For us, the description of service delivery is heard through the words and experiences of the administrators, the staff members, the collaborators, and the participants (clients). It is through their descriptions that a picture emerges of what they, as the respondents, consider to be those aspects that make these faith-based organizations and their programs unique and distinct from other social service agencies. The question remains to be answered as to whether these practices, in these settings, improves effectiveness.

DISCUSSION AND IMPLICATIONS

Our findings provide insight into how respondents from 15 programs across the United States see faith as influencing what they do. In summary, persons who are part of the religious traditions represented in this study are motivated by moral imperatives to serve and beliefs that they are accountable to God. Respondents' voices are similar in describing their calls to perform acts of service and to please God, even though the nuances of evangelical language differ. Tied to accountability to God are themes about the influence of mission on operations and the importance of founders, tradition and religious writings as ways of deeply embedding the traditions in the programmatic culture. These broad commonalities obscure differences in how overriding beliefs are carried out in practice. The data indicate that ways of being faith-based permeate service delivery in these programs, some ways being more manifest than others.

There are multiple implications of these findings for understanding human behavior in organizations, for professional social work practice, and for policy and research. Each is addressed below.

Implications for Understanding Human Behavior

Organizational culture theory reveals that there are deep underlying assumptions, expressed values, and artifacts in organizations (Schein, 1992). Underlying assumptions are so deeply ingrained that they may be driving what happens in organizations without anyone consciously recognizing it, although the program participants reveal that they recognize favorable practices and attitudes in the faith-based organizations that are elements that appeal to them in seeking services from these organizations (Yancey & Atkinson, 2004). Across roles (whether administration, staff, board, or client), the message about faith and its importance was similar from both the client and organizational perspective. Does this mean that all clients feel this way? Certainly not, but we have to keep in mind that clients were chosen by the agencies (not by us) and would likely reflect the views held by agency staff.

Values are expressions of what one believes, whereas artifacts are everything from behaviors to concrete religious symbols. It is these visibly expressive artifacts that have been the focus of typology development and of attempts to corral the faith-based dialogue–whether agencies can have religious pictures or figures on the walls or require clients to attend a religious event. Our findings indicate that in addition to artifacts, there are more fundamental elements in need of investigation. To fully capture faith-based programs, it is necessary to understand the assumptions underlying each program's expressed values of accountability to God and service. Only then will we understand what really motivates the persons who work and volunteer in these programs. Our findings are congruent with what Cnaan (1999) and his colleagues say about the importance of religion's "powerful and lasting effect on people's attitudes and behaviors" (p. 91) and their potential to motivate people to action.

Our findings, additionally, reveal that the underlying assumptions in faith-based programs do not necessarily come from an internal source (e.g., being embedded by a leader or founder) although they can be reinforced by human beings with deep faith. They often come from an external source that is filtered through the lens of each individual who interprets God's word, internalized into their own worldview. Therefore, there are multiple interpretations. The program that works appears to be one in which the persons who come together to deliver services find compatibility in their joint interpretations of how God's word is manifested. It is these joint interpretations that form the program's culture, even the organization's culture (e.g., Rogers et al., 2006). Founders certainly embed culture through their actions, but their motivations are from a higher external source.

Glickman (2002) adds insight to this finding, when he writes, "Each religious system, depending on its specific interpretation of the meaning of suffering, develops its own set of specific beliefs and behaviors" (p. 73). Indeed, specific beliefs and behaviors vary far more than descriptions of broader, overriding philosophies. Respondents reveal that one can serve God in multiple ways, even in contradictory ways. It is in these second-order, specific beliefs and behaviors, derived from the higher order basic assumptions and beliefs of service and accountability to God, on which we suspect the focus of the faith-based debate must move. To date, much of the faith-based initiatives and Charitable Choice debates have centered on what might be called third-order beliefs and behaviors–the visually-expressive elements of what one can see on a day-to-day basis in service providing programs (e.g., prayer, spiritual enrichment classes). We contend, however, that there is a middle ground between the higher-order beliefs and those visually expressive elements that warrant further exploration. This contention is supported by one writer (Warford, 2000) who states "Though often confused with belief, faith is actually something quite different. We can believe anything we want, and we often do, without necessarily ever having to demonstrate the truth of those beliefs. Faith, conversely, is fundamentally defined by the connection between what we profess to believe and what we actually do. It is consistency between belief and practice" (p. 5).

Our participants reveal this distinction between belief and faith in subtle ways that could be missed if one does not listen carefully. For example, respondents talked about the call from a higher being and tradition overriding other accountabilities such as those to government. The implication that if God's call is different from government's call, then God's call supercedes the secular accountability is not necessarily stated when respondents describe what makes their programs faith-based, but it is implied in their responses. If, for example, a highly evangelical group believes that God not only calls them to service but also mandates that the service must be performed in conjunction with converting souls, then the choice is to provide this service in an attempt to convert others. Otherwise, service will not be fully effective, according to God's desired outcomes. Similarly, if a faith-based tradition interprets God's call to mean that social service providers cannot give up on another person, no matter what that person does, then this has incredible consequences for how staff relate to clients. If one believes that there is always hope, that no one is hopeless, but that it may take a lifetime and that the future is open, then immediate outcomes may take on a lesser meaning as many agency or program boundary issues. If having tried one's best to serve is a motivator, then effort and process become more important than outcomes. One has been successful because one kept the faith, one has ministered, one has served, and the outcome may be one's own salvation as a result of having given it one's all. If one interprets God's word to mean that fathers must be reunited with their families, then this is not a program imperative; it is a God-given imperative. If one's tradition motivates a staff person to believe that one's life in the hereafter is dependent on the ability to respond to others' needs, then what one is able to do is tied to one's personal self-preservation and identity. This is much stronger than professional standards or government mandates. Thus, there is the potential for doing what needs to be done by any means necessary to achieve the higher calling, regardless of secular directives such as professional standards and best practices.

For many of these individuals in faith-based organizations, mission and accountability to God trumps secular or professional expectations. This finding is consistent with what Duncan and Stocks (2003) found in their study of 1200 pastors and internal control within their congregations. In terms of basic managerial systems (e.g., accounting, budgeting, and planning) in local churches "internal control is likely to be viewed as secular rather than sacred and, as a result, often considered irrelevant and unnecessary" (p. 221). Perhaps there are similar lessons to be learned in faith-based social service provision.

Implications for Professional Practice

Some administrators and staff members in this study had professional degrees in social work, nursing, and ministry. Others had dual degrees. Board members, collaborators, and clients were more likely to come from all walks of life with varied backgrounds. This is not unusual in community-based programs that deliver direct services. There is a mixture of volunteers, paraprofessional, and professional staff as well as number of persons playing dual roles (e.g., client and volunteer). Given this context, what are the implications for professional practice?

Practitioners involved in planning, administering, and delivering social services in local communities cannot escape the penetrating questions surrounding faith-based programming and the potential tensions that can arise when values clash. Even if they do not work directly in faith-based programs, they will have clients who are served by such programs or they will need to coordinate or collaborate with faith-based organizations in helping the poor and needy. It is incumbent upon practitioners to recognize the depth of motivation in long-established belief systems that drive these committed program staff and volunteers.

A lesson learned from respondents is just how deeply rooted faith can be. This is not surprising. What it underscores, however, is the fact that religious traditions are often so ingrained in a person's early development that they may override professional education and training introduced later in one's growth experience. Over and over, respondents explained that what they do is rooted in what they learned from early models, how they were taught as children, what they grew up with, and what they experienced in formative years when they were part of a long-established tradition. It may be that the socialization to religion in early childhood, which occurred far before they are socialized to professional values, motivates respondents to return to the roots of their faith to guide their actions. When one asks whom these respondents are trying to please, the answer is that it is God or some higher being. They actually talk about not needing recognition for what they do, almost as if recognition might somehow diminish their motivations. If an external force, internalized from early days, is a motivator, then the pressures of funders and the dictates of professional standards may seem of lesser importance than the calling by which one is inspired to provide social services to persons in need.

This raises incredible implications for the professional use of self in observing boundaries, minimizing potential risks inherent in playing multiple roles, and in not placing one's values on clients. Yet, depending on the faith tradition that respondents embraced, there were interviewees who felt it was their moral duty to witness their faith because they were ultimately accountable to God. There are persons providing services to clients who feel just as strongly that they must share their faith as part of their personal identity when their professional identity sees this as inherently unethical. Practitioners must be prepared to recognize how deep this commitment is because it cannot be countered by simply reminding a worker that this is not acceptable practice, when they fully believe that they are following through on moral standards perceived to be coming from God.

A major implication of our findings is that in teaching professionals about the various practices of diverse religious groups, we are only giving them the visible elements. While the expressed values of acts and faith are integral in the faith-based discussion, they do not tell the full story. The deep drivers of human behavior and practice are found in the specific beliefs and interpretations of individuals who are involved either as leaders or participants in faith-based organizations. The respondents in our study believe that helping the poor and needy will facilitate their becoming better Muslims, Jews, or Christians.

Implications for Policy and Research

The practices that emanate from being faith-based return us to the typology developed by Sider and Unruh (2004) in that they reflect the "value-expressive" elements that have been most controversial in the faith-based initiatives debates. One could argue that as long as those behavioral artifacts are kept in check that there is no superimposition of values on clients, residents, consumers, and other constituencies. However, we would argue that the ways of being faith-based are much more complicated than this. Without saying a word or engaging in an overt practice (e.g., prayer), interpretation of guiding philosophies are much deeper on a symbolic basis because they permeate every choice made, every option taken. These guiding philosophies are not only externally driven by a transcendent force, but they have been completely and developmentally internalized into the worldviews and sets of assumptions held by the persons who participate in the delivery of these programs.

The concepts of Charitable Choice and faith-based initiatives in the United States raised the nation's consciousness about the numerous and complex issues surrounding the use of public dollars by organizations that consider themselves to be based in faith. Numerous researchers across disciplines within the United States have risen to the challenge of studying various aspects of how congregations and religious nonprofits deliver human services to persons in need. The question of whether faith-based provision of services is somehow "better or not as good" as those services provided by secular organizations depends on which side of the political fence one sits. Critics of the current administration's "faith-based initiative" chide persons who enthusiastically portray the provision of services by various religious groups as being superior to those organizations that do not have religious ties. Conversely, proponents of faith-based delivery systems highlight any tidbits of research findings that appear to support their claims.

We are reminded of the dated debates in various sectors about whether for-profit organizations should deliver social services, based in dichotomous assumptions about their motives being either profit-driven or client-driven. Perhaps it is the focus on motives that undergirds the nature of faith-based delivery–perhaps the motives of secular providers cannot possibly parallel the motivation inspired by religious zeal. Whatever stand one takes, the questions asked and the inherent tensions in the debate are embedded in basic assumptions or worldviews that collide at the level of belief interpretation. A cadre of researchers and practitioners have joined forces to seek that illusive "faith factor" that makes a difference as if the question will be settled once and for all. We conclude that we have been focusing on artifacts because they are tangible. The deeper reality, however, is that the interpretation of beliefs form the assumptions that guide practice in faith-based organizations. If programs are offered in faith-based organizations, those "belief-based" assumptions permeate every choice made and every action taken.

If our findings are even somewhat reflective of what it means to work with faith-based programs, then how can the push for effectiveness-based programming be understood in this context? To answer this question one has to distinguish between quality and effectiveness-based measures. Quality measures are those that pertain to how people are treated, how they feel about the process of receiving service, and how the interactions of providers and participants are viewed. In the programs studied, quality is exceedingly high, according to our respondents. Effectiveness, on the other hand, asks whether a program works, does what it is supposed to do, and achieves its goals and objectives. Future research needs to examine the compatibility (or not) of secular and faith-based methods and measures of effectiveness. To study the effectiveness of faith-based organizations one must first unravel their distinctive foundations and components so that one can be able to find the relevant and unique variables to control for in identifying and using measurements that fit with what such programs can do. Hopefully, the study reported here begins that unraveling process.

CONCLUSION

In this grounded theory study, respondents were asked, "what makes your program faith-based?" As they provided examples of how faith influenced their thinking, behavior, and practice, a number of issues were raised. Human behavior in programs tied to faith is complicated by the relationship with a higher order, thus multiple accountabilities pertain. Professionals who are employed by, coordinate with, or make referrals to faith-based programs need to understand that the professional use of self in the worker-client relationship may not always be viewed the same, depending on one's faith tradition and what is acceptable in some organizational cultures. Implications for practice, policy, and research include the importance of recognizing that value-expressive elements are only the more visible artifacts of programmatic cultures. To study the effectiveness of faith-based organizations, researchers must first unravel the more subtle foundations and components that make them distinct. It is only in this way that relevant and unique faith-based variables can be manipulated and studied. Faith-based organizational and programmatic cultures may be inspired by deeply held religious belief systems that should not be neglected as we attempt to overcome the dearth of knowledge of the basic components of faith-based organizations.

REFERENCES

Billis, D. (1991). The roots of voluntary agencies: A question of choice. *Nonprofit and Voluntary Sector Quarterly, 20* (1), 57-69.

Brinckerhoff, P. C. (1999). *Faith-based management.* New York: John Wiley and Sons.

Cameron, K. S., & Quinn, R. E. (1999). *Diagnosing and changing organizational culture: Based on the competing values framework.* Reading, MA: Addision Wesley Longman, Inc.

Campbell, D. (2002). Outcomes assessment and the paradox of nonprofit accountability. *Nonprofit Management & Leadership, 12*(3), 243-259.

Chambre, S. M. (2001). The changing nature of "faith" in faith-based organizations: Secularization and ecumenism in four AIDS Organizations in New York City. *Social Service Review, 75,* 435-455.

Cnaan, R. A., Boddie, S.C., & Wineburg, J. (1999). *The newer deal: Social work and religion in partnership.* New York: Columbia University Press.

Duncan, J. B., & Stocks, M. H. (2003). The understanding of internal control principles of pastors. *Nonprofit Management & Leadership, 14*(2), 213-225.

Frost, P. J., Moore, L. F., Louis, M. R., Lundberg, C. C., & Martin, J. (1991). *Reframing organizational culture.* Newbury Park, CA: Sage.

Glaser, B. G., & Strauss, A. L. (1967). *The discovery of grounded theory.* Chicago: Aldine.

Goggin, M., & Orth, D. A. (2002). *How faith-based and secular organizations tackle housing for the homeless.* New York: The Roundtable on Religion and Social Welfare Policy.

Hasenfeld, Y. (2000). Social welfare administration and organizational theory (pp. 89-112). In R. J. Patti (Ed.). *The handbook of social welfare management.* Thousand Oaks, CA: Sage.

Holland, T. P., & Hester, D. C. (Eds.). (2000). *Building effective boards for religious organizations.* San Francisco, CA: Jossey-Bass.

Hyde, C. (2000). The hybrid nonprofit: An examination of feminist social movement organizations. *Journal of Community Practice, 8*(4), 45-67.

Jeavons, T. (1997). Identifying characteristics of 'religious' organizations: An exploratory proposal. In Demerarh, P. D. Hall, T. Schmitt, and R.H. Williams. *Sacred companies: Organizational aspects of religion and religious aspects of organizations,* pp. 79-95. New York: Oxford University Press.

Jeavons, T. (1992). When the management is the message: Relating values to management practice in nonprofit organizations. *Nonprofit Management & Leadership, 2*(4), 403-417.

Jeavons, T. H., & Basinger, R. B. (2000). *Growing givers hearts: Treating fundraising as ministry.* San Francisco, CA: Jossey-Bass.

Koroloff, N. M., & Briggs, H. E. (1996). The life cycle of family advocacy organizations. *Administration in Social Work, 20*(4), 23-42.

Lewis, D. (2002). Organization and management in the third sector: Toward a cross-cultural research agenda. *Nonprofit Management and Leadership, 13*(1), 67-83.

Martin, J. (2002). *Organizational culture: Mapping the terrain.* Thousand Oaks, CA: Sage.

Milofsky, C. (1997). Tradition. *Nonprofit and Voluntary Sector Quarterly, 26*(3), 261-268.

Minkoff, D.C. (2002). The emergence of hybrid organizational forms: Combining identity-based service provision and political action. *Nonprofit and Voluntary Sector Quarterly, 31*(3), 377-401

Monsma, S. (1996). *When sacred and secular mix: Religious nonprofit organizations and public money.* Lanham, MD: Rowman & Littlefield.

Netting, F. E., O'Connor, M. K., Thomas, M. L., & Yancey, G. (2005). Volunteers, staff, and participants: Mixing and phasing of roles in faith-based nonprofit programs. *Nonprofit and Voluntary Sector Quarterly, 34*(2), 179-205.

O'Connor, M. K. (2002). Using qualitative research in practice evaluation. Social workers' desk reference. (pp. 777-780). In: A. R. Roberts, and G. J. Greene. *Social Work Desk Reference.* New York: Oxford University Press.

Ott, J. S. (1989). *The organizational culture perspective.* Pacific Grove, CA: Brooks/ Cole.

Queen, E. L. II. (Ed.). (2000). *Serving those in need: A handbook for managing faith-based human service organizations.* San Francisco, CA: Jossey-Bass.

Quinn, R. E. (1988). *Beyond rational management.* San Francisco, CA: Jossey-Bass Publishers.

Rogers, R., Yancey, G., Singletary, J., Garland, D., & Brennan Homiak, K. (2006). Faith identity and faith culture: New empirical dimensions for understanding congregations and religiously-affiliated organizations. Retrieved January 6, 2006 from http://bayloruniversityschoolofsocialwork/cfcm/faithidentityandfaithculture

Salamon, L. M. (Ed.). (2002). *The state of nonprofit America.* Washington, DC: Brookings Institution Press.

Schein, E. H. (1992). *Organizational culture and leadership* (2nd ed.). San Francisco: Jossey-Bass.

Schultz, M. (1995). *On studying organizational cultures: Diagnosis and understanding.* New York: Walter de Gruyter.

Sider, R. J., & Unruh, H. R. (2004). Typology of religious characteristics of social service and educational organizations and programs. *Nonprofit and Voluntary Sector Quarterly, 33*(1), 109-134.

Stoesen, L. (July, 2004). Collaborating with faith-based services. *NASW NEWS, 49*(7), (p. 4).

Strauss, A., & Corbin, J. (1998). *Basics of qualitative research: Techniques and procedures for developing grounded theory.* Thousand Oaks, CA: Sage.

Warford, M. L. (2000). Stewards of hope. In T. P. Holland & D. C. Hester (Eds.). *Building effective boards for religious organizations* (pp. 3-23). San Francisco, CA: Jossey-Bass.

Weiss, R. S. (1994). *Learning from strangers: The art and method of qualitative interview studies.* New York: Free Press.

Wineburg, B. (2001). *A limited partnership: The politics of religion, welfare, and social service.* New York: Columbia University Press.

Wosh, P. J. (2004). *Covenant house: Journey of a faith-based charity.* Philadelphia: University of Pennsylvania Press.

Yancey, G., & Atkinson, K. (2004). The impact of caring in faith-based organizations: What participants say. *Social Work & Christianity, 31*(3), 254-266.

Concluding Remarks:
Common Findings and Challenges

Stephanie C. Boddie
Ram A. Cnaan

One can observe based on the reported studies in this volume that two conclusions have emerged. First, from a societal point of view, we have not invested nearly enough in assessing the effectiveness of faith-based social services. The empirical studies reported here, and a handful of others, all suggest that we are in the infancy stage of faith-based program evaluation. The methodologies used by the pioneering empirical researchers in this area fall very short of the challenges posed by the scholars in the first part of this volume. The sums of money available for this kind of research are meager, and hence there has hardly been a chance to utilize the many sophisticated designs proposed in the first part of the volume. Before any conclusive statements can be made regarding the effectiveness of faith-based organizations, many more studies are needed and generous funds are required. The researchers who went ahead and made some progress in the puzzle should be commended for their heroic efforts and important findings. However, much more resources are needed for future research, and we are many years away from any authoritative or comprehensive answers.

Second, our tentativeness about conclusive results notwithstanding, it seems safe to suggest that faith-based organizations as a whole are neither superior nor inferior to their secular counterparts. It seems that

[Haworth co-indexing entry note]: "Concluding Remarks: Common Findings and Challenges." Boddie, Stephanie C., and Ram A. Cnaan. Co-published simultaneously in *Journal of Religion & Spirituality in Social Work* (The Haworth Pastoral Press, an imprint of The Haworth Press, Inc.) Vol. 25, No. 3/4, 2006, pp. 287-291; and: *Faith-Based Social Services: Measures, Assessments, and Effectiveness* (ed: Stephanie C. Boddie, and Ram A. Cnaan) The Haworth Pastoral Press, an imprint of The Haworth Press, Inc., 2006, pp. 287-291

overall they achieve equal results to secular providers. However, their net contribution may be in lowering the cost and enhancing competition in the field as a whole, but even this is understudied. Competition is perceived as an advantage for cost-cutting options (McNabb, 2005). Participating in the bidding process for public contracts to provide social services may by itself increase efficiency and reduce costs as new competitors force old competitors to lower costs and be more effective or they will lose their advantage (Dixit, 2005). It should be noted that faith-based providers are closer to the recipients of the services than are public civil servants and therefore tend to have better information about local needs; furthermore, they also experience some direct benefits from these actions and will therefore perform them for lower salaries and/or weaker incentive payments. In addition, a large part of the service cost may be subsidized by the faith community (using volunteers and sacred space) and their overall cost may be lower per outcome unit than that of secular congregations, but again, this needs further study.

Clients, regardless of "real" progress, seem to like faith-based social service workers and see them as more nurturing and more caring when compared with public providers. This finding is strongly evident in the Monsma and the Sinha studies, but also coincides with other studies. For example, Goggin and Orth (2002) found among New York City homeless people who lost welfare eligibility that in many cases the clients made explicit references to their relationships with frontline faith-based workers, describing them as "dedicated," "nurturing," "caring," "helping," and "loving" (p. 46). These authors, however, caution us that not all faith-based social services were characterized as such, but still many more than the secular ones.

As noted earlier, the studies also show that one of the key barriers to successful assessment of effectiveness is state politics. Due to the emphasis on state sovereignty embedded in the "new federalism" ideology, comparing states is difficult unless the agencies studied are independent of the state, such as in the case of a provider contracting directly with the federal government. However, even within one state, changing policies over time makes longitudinal studies impossible as some clients are terminated when their sources of support dry out. Also, making comparisons within states is difficult when various counties pass different regulations.

Furthermore, as Sinha aptly demonstrated, good intentions of service providers to help in research efforts are often confronted by lack of administrative know-how and lack of resources. This, in itself, does not mean that the service provided is of a lesser quality. Often this is not the case. This issue is extremely important in an environment of very limited resources for effectiveness research. Bielefeld and Sinha, among others, strongly demonstrated that over-stretched staff members cannot be relied upon to carry out data collection for evaluation research and that more often than not, they will fail in routine data collection at the expense of responding to a client real crisis. Many faith-based service providers are working to their full capacity, as staff members are often already over-utilized and there is almost nothing more they can do. Put differently, if anything breaks or if a crisis arises, there is a very small margin for adaptation. One could see it as a sign of efficiency, but one could also see it as a sign of low ability to react to arising crises or changes. Nevertheless, many of our contributors were able to carry out their research because they save on costs by relying on the service providers to assist in data collection. Future studies should avoid this potential pitfall by hiring research assistants who can be placed at the service agencies and will be a reliable source of data collection.

The studies in this volume did not find any indications of coerced or even implied proselytism. It seems that this is a small issue regarding the faith-based initiatives. It could be that the first wave of public fund recipients did not dare evangelize as they knew that they were under close scrutiny. However, it is also possible that they knew that clients dislike forced religion. For example, Sager and Stephens (2005, p. 297) studied a set of homeless shelters where sermons and prayers were part of the social care (these were not part of the faith-based initiative) and concluded that "regardless of their religious beliefs, two thirds of the homeless respondents reacted negatively to the sermons they heard at congregation-based food programs, characterizing them as coercive, hypocritical, condescending, and conflicting with their own beliefs." These authors suggested that the relevant clergy failed to understand the particular world of the homeless people. But there is an alternate explanation: perhaps congregations provide services in order to solidify the members within; perhaps there is really no intention to solicit new members from among the homeless, and there is no assumption that one material service can transform a person's worldview and beliefs (Cnaan, Boddie, Handy, Yancey, & Schneider, 2002).

The findings from this volume also suggest four key domains that require attention in future effectiveness assessment studies concerning faith-based organizations. The first domain is the classification of religious or spiritual content of programs (including programs identified as secular) and the extent of the content. It is clear that not all faith-based organizations perceive faith in a similar vein, and they may also differ in how much faith should be interwoven into the service delivery. Although some good models have been developed in this regard (see review in Cnaan, Kang, McGrew, & Sinha, 2003; Unruh & Sider, 2005), there is still a need for an easy to use yet reliable measure of an organization's religiosity and its impact on service delivery.

Second, just as these faith-based organizations are not the same in their inclusion of theology into their daily practice (religious integration) they are also diverse on many other organizational aspects. The literature about organization effectiveness includes discussion of experience, size, budget and other factors that may account to success regardless of the sector identification. As Goggin and Orth (2001) noted in a study of housing services in Grand Rapids, MI that there is no standard approach to service delivery that characterizes all FBOs in a certain industry (field of service) as there are significant differences among FBOs. Some are more sophisticated organizationally while others are not. It is important to take the next step in developing frameworks for sorting out these organizational differences.

Third, there is a need for the specification of outcome variables. As Thyer, von Furstenberg, and Grettenberger and her colleagues suggested, we have a very rough and imprecise vocabulary of outcome measures in social services in general and in faith-based social services in particular. It is important for the research community to come up with clear outcome measures so that rigorous studies will be accepted without debates about what was actually measured. In this respect, Fischer and Stelter's ideas of adopting outcome measurement practices currently used within the nonprofit sector may be of value.

Fourth, in many studies, both client and staff follow-up suffered from high attrition rates. There are numerous statistical methods to help us analyze the data of participant attrition in empirical studies. However, when a large number of providers leave and many clients oscillate between programs, both the internal and external validity of findings are threatened.

In summary, this volume has started a new voyage. While the rhetoric about faith-based social services is rampant, actual empirical studies and discussion regarding the most appropriate topics and means of study are still long-term endeavors. It is possible that we will never know complete answers to our questions, but we are obliged to keep trying to rationalize the sphere of public service delivery with the use of tax-payer money. We hope that this volume will galvanize the effort to scientifically study religious services.

REFERENCES

Cnaan, R. A., Kang, J. J., McGrew, C. C., & Sinha, J. W. (2003). Identiteit meetbaar maken: Gedachten van de andere kant van de Atlantische Oceaan (Incorporating religious identity into organizational identity: Thoughts from the other side of the Atlantic ocean). *Bulletib Onderwijs & Inspiratie, 32* (5), 23-25.

Dixit, A. (2005). Incentive contracts for faith-based organizations to deliver social services. In S. Lahiri and P. Maiti (Eds.). *Economic theory in a changing world: Policy modeling for growth.* New Delhi: Oxford University Press. Retrieved December 2, 2005 from: http://www.princeton.edu/~dixitak/home/faith.pdf

Goggin, M. L., & Orth, D. A. (2002). *How faith-based and secular organizations tackle housing for the homeless.* Albany, NY: University of New York at Albany, the Rockefeller Institute of Government.

McNabb, M. L. (2005). Gatekeeping between government and religion: Faith-based initiative competition and supervision. Retrieved December 2, 2005 from: http://shepherdapps.wlu.edu/pdf/mcnabb423_03.pdf

Sager, R., & Stephens, L. S. (2005). Clients' reactions to religious elements at congregation-run feeding establishments. *Nonprofit and Voluntary Sector Quarterly, 34,* 297-315.

Unruh, H. R., & Sider, R. J. (2005). Saving souls, serving society: Understanding the faith Factor in church-based social ministry. New York: Oxford University Press.

Index